ADHD Brains Don't Come In One Size

A Realistic Guide to Understanding Adult ADHD and Finding What Works for You

Amy Harper

To my family, whose unwavering love guides me in all that I do—thank you for being my steady light in life's stormy moments.

Preface

Dear Reader,

Thank you for choosing "ADHD Brains Don't Come In One Size." It means a lot to me that you're joining me on this journey.

ADHD has been a part of my life since I was a child. I've had my ups and downs for as long as I can remember. And just like you, I've faced many challenges in my professional and personal life.

Despite all the difficulties, I've learned invaluable lessons. I've spent years trying to make sense of ADHD and figure out how to thrive with it. During my decades working in the field of psychology, I've met and helped so many people like you.

This book isn't just about theory. Its purpose is to share real-life experiences, practical tips, and exercises to help you better understand your brain and develop personalized strategies so you can thrive in different aspects of your life.

Whether you're newly diagnosed or have been navigating ADHD for years, this book is for you. I hope you achieve your goals!

Amy Harper

Exclusive Offer

Thank you for purchasing this book! Before we get started, I would like you to know that I am committed to helping you thrive with ADHD. Because of that, I am offering you this exclusive offer, which is optional and only complimentary to the contents of this book, in case you want to walk the extra mile.

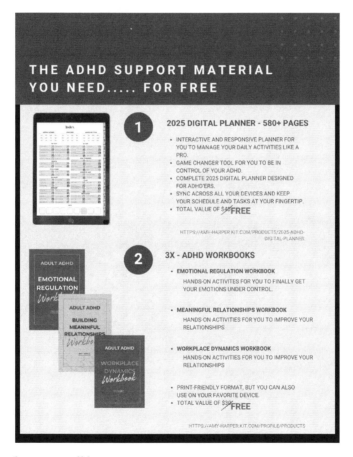

This is what you will have access to:

1) 2025 Digital Planner: A responsive planner for you to use in your pre-ferred annotation app. Keep your calendar, to-do lists, checklists, guides, and so much more at your fingertips. This is a tool for your daily use.

2) ADHD Workbooks: This package includes **three workbooks** to give you a hands-on experience while reading this book: Emotional Regulation Workbook, Building Meaningful Relationships Workbook and Workplace Dynamics Workbook. These are optional companions to "ADHD Brains Don't Come in One Size" because they relate to the content you are about to read. You may print them or use them digitally.

These products are available for sale in my store, but I am offering them for free to you. I want you to be equipped and feel confident about the journey you are about to start.

Scan the QR code below to get access to all of them.

(https://amy-harper.kit.com/fca05047ec)

Contents

Introduction

Why This Book Matters

"The treatment tools that work for ADHD are comparatively easy to acquire. It is hard, though, to undo the years of harsh and unhelpful feedback to which a person with ADHD has been exposed."

ADDitudemag

Have you ever had one of those dreams where you're trying to run away from something or someone, and your legs simply refuse to work? Or worse, you try to scream, but no sound escapes your mouth? Well, that's kind of what it feels like to function as an ADHDer in a world created for neurotypicals; no matter how hard you try or how desperate you are to move forward, you're stuck in place. Unfortunately, most non-ADHDers don't see it this way, so they give advice like "just focus" or "just stop procrastinating," which is about as helpful as telling a visually impaired person to "just see."

At the other end of the spectrum, ADHDers are served with books and resources that promise magical transformation. They provide tools and techniques that claim to hold all the answers to *curing* your ADHD and making you function like a neurotypical. But let's be real for a second: Those books ain't going to work, my friend. How do I know? Because

I've tried them, many, many, many of them, and the only thing that transformed was my inner peace into pure frustration!

If that sounds familiar, you're exactly where you need to be.

Because here's the truth: you're not lazy, you're not broken, and you don't need more willpower. ADHD isn't about *knowing* what to do—it's about *getting yourself to do it.* And that's the frustrating part, right? You know exactly what needs to be done, yet somehow, the dishes stay undone, the emails pile up, and you're running late... again.

If you've ever felt stuck in that cycle, you're not alone. And you're not doomed to stay there.

Why This Book Exists

Growing up, I knew my brain worked a little differently than most of my friends. While their backpacks were organized and clean, I often found forgotten permission slips and old sandwiches at the bottom of mine. Every new year, I would promise myself that this year would be different. I had goals to remember to do homework (or remember to at least write it down in my diary and actually check the diary when I got home). I had plans to be the most organized student in class, but it never lasted long. All the things that came so naturally to my friends seemed impossible to me. At first, I just assumed I was forgetful. But as time went on, I started to realize that no matter how hard I tried to be 'better,' my brain refused to cooperate. Even after I received my diagnosis at a young age, I drew my own conclusion: There's something wrong with me, and I am a failure.

It was only later in life, when I started researching the ADHD mind, that I understood a fundamental truth: I'm not a failure. I'm simply a cactus being asked to live in the rainforest. Since then, I've dedicated my career to understanding the human mind, both physically and psychologically, so I can help ADHDers thrive in a world that isn't set up for us. That's why I believe this book is different from most other ADHD books on the market: I get you, and I get your mind. I *actually* get it.

But what's the difference between conventional ADHD resources (and resources created by neurotypicals) and solutions that work for the ADHD mind? The fundamental differences are flexibility, adaptability, and personalization. However, even small things like the tone of voice, the depth of the advice provided, and the use of science can make a huge difference in the effectiveness of the advice provided.

So what exactly makes the difference between an ADHD-friendly strategy and one that sets you up for failure? Let's break it down.

	Conventional ADHD resources	This book
Tone	Overly optimistic or overly technical	Brutally honest, empathetic, and a dash of magical humor
Content depth	Focuses on surface-level tips without exploring the root of the problem	Deep dive into ADHD's neurological and behavioral aspects
Flexibility	One-size-fits-all approach	Adaptable strategies tailored to diverse ADHD needs
Scientific basis	Limited or no references to credible research	Backed by studies with citations for further exploration
Reader engagement	Dense text that's difficult (and boring) to read	Bite-size insights, anecdotes, and visual aids (like this one)

Table 1: Differences between conventional ADHD resources and this book.

With all of this in mind, here's what I can promise you about this book:

- I won't pretend as if ADHD is something you can fix, nor will I pretend it's a superpower—because it's not.

- I'll keep it real and honest, focusing on techniques you can adjust and adapt to fit your specific needs.

- We won't just scratch the surface but take a deep dive into understanding the ADHD mind.

- I'll keep it short, to the point, and won't bore you to sleep.

How to Get the Most Out of This Book

So, will this book change your life? It can, if you're willing to take the tools and make them your own. ADHD doesn't have a one-size-fits-all solution. Instead, I can provide you with the foundations of brilliant techniques you can build on to ensure they work for you. But you'll have to put in the work. If you want to see real change, I encourage you to experiment, take notes, and try things out. Some strategies will work for you, and some won't—and that's the point. ADHD isn't about finding the *perfect* system, but about *building your own toolkit* of strategies that fit your life.

There will be moments where you might feel resistant, frustrated, or doubtful. That's normal. But keep going. ADHD isn't about willpower—it's about understanding your brain and making things easier, not harder.

If you've ever felt like every ADHD solution out there works for everyone—except you—this book is for you. If you've ever felt like ADHD advice doesn't take into account your *actual* reality, this book is for you.

But first you need to have a clear and deep understanding of ADHD and what is really going on inside your mind, so that's where we'll start in Chapter One.

Are you ready to jump in and get started? I know, probably not. So, go ahead, grab your comfort blanket, your water bottle, and your forgotten cup of coffee, and set aside the next 20 minutes to begin this journey. If, after 20 minutes, you've been pulled into a hyperfocus, feel free to keep going. But don't put too much pressure on yourself to finish this book in one sitting. If you do stop after a couple of minutes, remember to keep the book somewhere you'll see it or be reminded to come back to it. Otherwise, we both know you'll forget it ever existed (I told you, I get it!). Most importantly, have fun getting to know your mind better!

Chapter 1

Understanding ADHD at a Deeper Level

"Everybody is a genius. But if you judge a fish by its ability to climb a tree, it will live its whole life believing that it is stupid."
Albert Einstein

When you read "Understanding ADHD at a Deeper Level," how do you feel? You're probably one of the following two people: You're either excited about learning more and making understanding ADHD your latest hyper-fixation, or you don't really care and want to jump straight to the practical techniques and methods. Either way, you're welcome here to be as excited or uninterested as you are. But if you're the latter, perhaps I can entice you with this: The better you understand ADHD, the more effective the later tools and techniques will be. I'm not in the business of making you sit through a science lecture purely for the sake of creating content. Instead, I want to teach you the science of what's happening up there in your unique mind because it will add value to your life.

Understanding ADHD at a deeper level is more than just gaining knowledge. It's about getting to know yourself. Let me tell you a little story, I have a friend who is a marine biologist, and you can often find her deep-sea diving with sharks and other marine life. But when she started her career, she started with textbooks and studies. She knew that in order to be safe and help the marine life, she had to understand them first. She couldn't just jump into the water on day one and hope for the best. She had to prepare. She spent months learning their behaviors, understanding how they react to movement, and even practicing in controlled environments before ever setting foot in open water. By the time she finally dove in, she wasn't just knowledgeable—she was ready.

While you and I might not be marine biologists or planning on swimming with sharks, we need to understand our minds first before jumping straight into methods and techniques. So, use that as your motivation to take a closer look at this chapter, allowing your curious mind to learn more about yourself. To understand ADHD, we need to explore the different archetypes of the brain, including the wanderer, the doer, the switchboard operator, the emotional amplifier, and the messengers.

The Default Mode Network: The Wanderer

The default mode network (DMN) is an interconnected group of brain structures, including the prefrontal cortex, posterior cingulate cortex, and the inferior parietal lobule (Brandman et al., 2021). The concept of the DMN was first developed after researchers found that the brains of test subjects were active even when they weren't doing anything. They weren't trying to solve a puzzle or communicate with someone else; they were simply doing nothing, yet their brains were active. This begged the question: with what? This led researchers to discover that certain parts of the brain are still active even when you are resting (*Know Your Brain: Default Mode Network*, n.d.).

What Does the DMN Do?

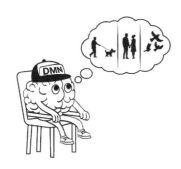 The DMN is nicknamed the wanderer because it's what happens when your mind wanders off. Even when you're relaxing and not busy with anything, your mind will begin to wander away. Sometimes, this leads to reflecting on your day or a conversation you had earlier, while for others, the mind begins to create stories or pictures. For many, this is when planning kicks in, and you're creating a long mental to-do list. Let's take a closer look at what the wanderer is in charge of.

Reflection

Refection occurs when you think deeply and carefully about something. It involves looking back on experiences, events, or ideas, examining each from a different angle. For this reason, reflection can be a very valuable tool for growth as it allows you to see things from a new point of view. It's the act of reflection that encourages you to learn from mistakes and make improvements (HCPC, 2021). Reflection occurs during DMN when you don't have to think of anything else and can allow your mind to process information it already received earlier. It also allows the brain to draw connections between different ideas, allowing you to come up with new solutions for problems.

Imagination

The DMN is also in charge of your imagination. Have you ever closed your eyes to have a quick rest, and suddenly, there's a whole new movie playing in your mind? Well, that's your imagination doing its thing when there's nothing else to focus on. The DMN plays a crucial role in imagination, particularly in constructing and evaluating imagined scenarios. Studies have shown that the DMN is active when individuals engage in tasks that involve imagining future events, such as daydreaming or planning (Mancuso et al., 2022). The DMN also controls the vividness of your imagination, making your daydreaming a tad bit more realistic, allowing you to experience emotions based on a mental image.

Planning

Lastly, the wanderer helps the human mind to make plans by envisioning future scenarios and tasks since it's not actively busy with a particular task. This allows the brain to process information and form new connections between ideas. The DMN is also connected to the limbic system, which is the part of the brain responsible for emotions. Due to this connection, the DMN can play a role in your emotions and how you're feeling about a possible future event after playing the scenario in your mind (Ramsøy, 2024).

The wanderer seems like a pretty nice character to take up residence in your mind, right? For most neurotypical people, yes. Why? Because the DMN works exactly as we just described it. But that's not necessarily the case when it comes to ADHD.

How Does ADHD Affect the DMN?

In an ADHD mind, the DMN is way more active than in other minds. You know that constant and familiar pull demanding that you pay attention to anything but the task at hand? Well, that's thanks to the DMN. The DMN contributes to ADHDers making mistakes due to a lack of concentration and focus. It's what makes us look careless when we struggle to focus on the task right in front of us or begin to zone out when someone else is talking. More specifically, ADHD and DMN together often lead to the following two issues.

Intrusive Thoughts

Intrusive thoughts are those unwanted, unplanted, and often disturbing thoughts that pop into your might unexpectedly. They can range from mild annoyances to severe obsessions about literally anything. In some cases, intrusive thoughts can be violent, sexual, or socially unacceptable, while, in other instances, they can include worries about being embarrassed in public or doubting whether you've locked the door (Seif & Winston, 2018). The ADHD mind can influence the DMN to think intrusive thoughts. This is due to your DMN being overactive, creating links between thoughts where there aren't any, and prompting your mind to think of *random* things even when you have something else to focus on. Instead of the DMN running wild while you're resting or not busy with anything, in an ADHD mind, it might interrupt what you're doing to drop an intrusive thought on you (Posner et al., 2015).

Procrastination

ADHD and the DMN can also lead to procrastination. Procrastination happens when you delay or postpone a task or a set of tasks. While procrastination is common for most people, it increases in frequency and severity with someone who has ADHD. Why? Because of an overactive DMN, it is hard to control thoughts. Instead, it will feel like you're stuck in limbo and unable to do the task at hand. Your mind will provide you with all sorts of other things to entertain you and keep you busy, preventing you from doing the task at hand (*Default Mode Network vs Task*, 2024).

Because of an overactive DMN, every task feels like rolling a boulder up a hill for someone with ADHD. Just when you think you've made progress, the boulder slips, forcing you to start all over again. The overactive DMN almost becomes like the bully on the playground—loud, intrusive, and refusing to wait its turn. It shoves its way in, dominating every mental space, while the other friend—the task-positive network—stands on the sidelines, waiting for a chance to play but constantly being pushed out of the game.

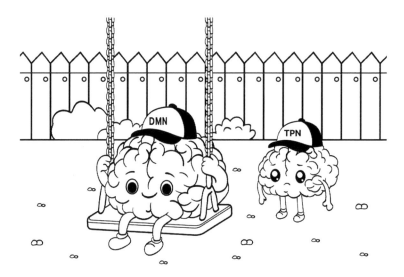

The Task-Positive Network: The Doer

The task-positive network (TPN) is the DMN's counterpart. In other words, it's your brain's work mode, responsible for getting things done. It's when you're focused on something and not in rest mode. The TPN involves a variety of functions, including working memory, decision-making, and problem-solving. The TPN is what pushes us to be goal-oriented and focused. It allows you to ignore distractions and remain focused on the task or goal at hand. Let's take a closer look at what exactly the TPN is in charge of.

What Does the TPN Do?

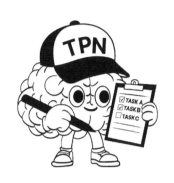

The TPN is nicknamed the doer because it gets things done. It's that one friend in every group who always gets stuff done no matter how busy they are. They might be working the longest hours, but they're still the ones showing up with dinner or planning the friend-getaway. While the TPN is working hard and in the driver's seat, the DMN takes a back-seat and relaxes. In most cases, the DMN listens and patiently waits for its turn to have a go at running the mind. While the DMN is chilling, the TPN is responsible for focus, problem-solving, and productivity.

Focus

The TPN is the brain's command center for attention and goal-directed behavior. When you need to concentrate on a task, the TPN jumps into motion (Hamilton et al., 2011). It allows you to focus by filtering any distractions and tuning out irrelevant information that might pull your attention away. This allows for steady focus and attention. Part of the focus is also maintaining and sustaining the effort of focus. Whether it's studying for an exam, writing a report, or simply following a recipe, the TPN helps us sustain our mental effort over time and prevents our minds from wandering (Orman, 2024).

Problem-Solving

The TPN plays a major role in problem-solving by facilitating focused attention, cognitive control, and the manipulation of information. When faced with a challenge, the TPN springs into action, directing our mental resources toward analyzing the problem, identifying relevant information, and generating potential solutions (Boyatzis et al., 2014). One of the key ways the TPN contributes to problem-solving is by enhancing working memory, such as memorizing a combination of numbers for a few minutes before you can write it down. Working memory is essential for evaluating different approaches to certain situations as it allows us to temporarily hold and manipulate information in our minds. The TPN strengthens this process, enabling us to keep track of multiple pieces of information simultaneously and shift our focus between different aspects of the problem (Dixon, 2022).

Productivity

When engaged in a task, the TPN begins to allocate resources and coordinate neural activity to ensure smooth and effective performance. This function, combined with the TPN's ability to filter out irrelevant information, is essential for achieving goals and completing projects efficiently. By suppressing distracting thoughts and impulses, the TPN allows us to channel our mental energy towards the desired outcome. The TPN is also involved in higher-level cognitive processes, such as planning and decision-making (Boyatzis et al., 2014).

How Does ADHD Affect the TPN?

The ADHD mind has an overactive DMN, so what does that mean for the TPN? We already said the DMN can be a bit of a bully, which means that the TPN doesn't always get to *do* what it's supposed to do. Instead, it gets interrupted by the DMN and pushed away from the control room. In neurotypical individuals, these networks function in a complementary manner: when one is active, the other is suppressed. However, in individuals with ADHD, this balance is disrupted (*Default Mode Network vs Task*, 2024). An underactive TPN can lead to these two issues:

Task Initiation Issues

When there is a task at hand that needs to be done, the TPN is supposed to take over. But what happens when the DMN refuses to give up control? Well, you'll end up unable to start the task at hand because it will feel impossible. Your mind will distract you with other thoughts instead of pushing you to get the task done. The persistent DMN activity leads to a constant stream of internal thoughts, making it very hard to focus on anything clearly. This can result in daydreaming and wandering, distracting you from initiating the task you are aware of. Furthermore, the DMN can also make you feel overwhelmed by the task at hand since the TPN didn't take over and provide you with the energy and focus you need to accomplish the task (*Default Mode Network vs Task*, 2024).

Short Focus Span – Or, Sometimes, Too Much Focus?

Since the DMN doesn't want to give up control and allow the TPN to work, it results in a very short attention and focus span. The DMN steps back for a short while, and during that time, the TPN thrives, resulting in good attention and focus. However, as soon as the DMN takes back control and pushes TPN away, the focus and attention are broken. This is what happens within the ADHD mind and why you're struggling to pay attention and focus on something for a long period of time. While it might come easily for neurotypicals who don't have overactive DMNs, for ADHDers, paying attention is really challenging.

But here's where it gets weird: sometimes, instead of struggling to focus, you can't seem to stop focusing—even when you want to. This is hyperfocus, a state where the TPN locks in so intensely that the DMN, instead of interrupting, gets completely shut out. Think of it like the DMN getting booted off the playground, leaving the TPN to run the show with no supervision. While this can be helpful for deep work or creativity, it's also why ADHDers can spend five hours tweaking a spreadsheet but can't start a five-minute task. Hyperfocus is another example of ADHD being less about "attention deficit" and more about attention dysregulation—the brain struggles to find balance between too much focus and not enough.

This begs the question: who is allowing the DMN to bully the TPN? Isn't there a teacher we can call when DMN is hogging the playground? Well, that's the job of the salience network. Also known as the switchboard operator.

The Salience Network: The Switchboard Operator

The salience network has many names. In some studies, it's referred to as the midcingulo-insular network (M-CIN), while others refer to it as the ventral attention network. I like to call the switchboard operator since it's in charge of detecting and responding to important internal and external stimuli (Seeley, 2019). The salience network (SN) constantly monitors the environment and internal bodily sensations. Based on the information gathered by monitoring, it also decides what deserves our attention and how to react to certain stimuli.

Let's say you're walking down the street when suddenly there's a loud noise. The salience network quickly alerts the other brain networks that something has happened and decides whether to prompt the fight or flight system or whether to write it off as nothing to be concerned about. It's like your body's 911 operator. Whatever information it receives, it decides who to dispatch to take care of the problem. When you're feeling hungry, for example, the salience network signals the need to address these internal needs, prompting you to think of food and decide to eat something.

How Does ADHD Affect the Salience Network?

In a neurotypical mind, the switchboard operator effectively controls when the DMN should be active or when it's time for a TPN moment. It switches between the two based on your needs and surroundings. If you're writing a test, it will switch the charge to TPN, but when you're daydreaming on the bus, it will switch to DMN. This results in effective focus, attention, and imagination when it's needed. Unfortunately, it's not that simple in the ADHD mind. For ADHDers, the salience network is often disrupted, leading to several characteristic symptoms, including the following two.

Getting Stuck in DMN

In an ADHD mind, the salience network is like a lazy teacher who knows they should be doing rounds in the playground to ensure that everyone gets a turn on the swings but instead is resting in the breakroom with a cup of coffee. However, when they finally patrol the grounds, they tell the kid who just got onto the swing that it's time to give someone else a turn. In other words, they're a little out of touch and not fully aware of what's happening. In the same way, the salience network in an ADHD mind is less effective at filtering out irrelevant information and prioritizing important stimuli. This often leads to getting stuck in DMN and ignoring the TPN (Orman, 2024).

What does that mean for you and me? It means we're more likely to have wandering minds even when we're busy with tasks, and we're way more likely to get distracted by things other people don't seem to notice (like that annoying lawnmower nagging in your ear while you're trying to listen to what your boss is saying).

Overexerting the TPN

Since the switchboard operator isn't as vigilant as it should be, it often allows distractions to run wild without limits. Instead of filtering out the noise and things that aren't important, it will tell your mind that it's something to pay attention to. This usually occurs while the TPN is working (when you're focusing on someone or something). As a result, your TPN has to work way harder to remain focused. Imagine walking on a narrow bridge, carrying an important message to the person on the other side of the bridge. You have to focus on getting there, not fall off, and remember the message, right? Well, now imagine someone blasting an air horn, throwing water balloons at you, and singing that annoying jingle you can never get out of your head. Technically, you still have the same task as before, but it's suddenly much, much harder to achieve!

In other words, when the switchboard operator allows more noise and distractions, the TPN has to work harder to accomplish a very simple task, leading to overexertion. That's why tasks that seem simple to neurotypicals can be incredibly challenging and exhausting for an ADHDer. However, we can't blame everything on the salience network. It's not the only one in charge, after all. The limbic system also plays a significant role, especially in how you react and respond to emotions.

The Limbic System: The Emotional Amplifier

The limbic system is another system that runs the risk of overexertion. What exactly is it? It's a complex network of brain structures located deep within the brain, beneath the cerebral cortex, and it includes the amygdala, hippocampus, hypothalamus, and nucleus accumbens. The limbic system has a few important roles, especially when it comes to emotional regulation. The limbic system is in the driver's seat of emotions, processing and regulating feelings such as fear, anger, joy, and sadness. It helps us make sense of our emotions and how to respond appropriately. It takes cues from others as well as from internal messaging in order to decide what we're feeling, why we're feeling it, and how we should respond (Torrico & Abdijadid, 2019).

Another important task of the limbic system is forming and consolidating memories associated with emotions. This allows the mind to learn from past experiences and adapt to future environments with the same emotional triggers. In other words, if you had an awful argument with your loved one because of something that was said or done, your limbic system will process it and remember that it happened. So, next time you're in a similar spot, you'll know that if you were to say or do that same thing again, it will most likely erupt into another argument.

In essence, the limbic system is essential for our emotional, social, and cognitive well-being, as it helps us to navigate the world around us, understand and respond to our emotions, and learn and grow from our experiences (*What is the limbic system?*, 2024).

How Does ADHD Affect the Limbic System?

In an ADHD mind, the limbic system is a bit of an overachiever and works overtime. However, instead of overtime leading to more effective tasks, it can lead to amplified emotions and poor emotional regulation. In other words, the smallest emotional shift might send the entire limbic system into panic mode, resulting in feeling way more intense emotions than what the situation actually requires. That's why ADHDers often experience extreme mood swings or get irritated by small things. There are two specific ways in which ADHD affects the limbic system, so let's have a look.

Overactive Amygdala

The amygdala is part of the limbic system and is responsible for processing emotions such as fear and anxiety. However, in an ADHD mind, the amygdala is overly sensitive, leading to heightened emotional reactivity. This leads to increased feelings of fear and anxiety in everyday situations that aren't objectively threatening. Something fairly harmless might seem much more terrifying or dangerous than it actually is—like a simple phone call might feel frightening. This can also lead to emotional outbursts, especially outbursts of anger, sadness, and frustration.

Weakened Regulation

The limbic system, or as I like to call it, the emotional amplifier, can also be affected by ADHD in the way it regulates bodily functions that are connected to the stress response. In other words, when you have ADHD, your limbic system will have a harder time managing stress, leading to higher levels of cortisol (the stress hormone). In turn, this contributes to sleep disturbances and increased impulsivity (sounds familiar?). This is a result of poor communication between the limbic system and the prefrontal cortex, making it harder to calm intense emotions.

But why is there poor communication between the limbic system and other parts of the brain? Is the problem with the one sending the message or the one receiving it? Perhaps both, or perhaps it's neither. In fact, a lot of these issues are a result of the messengers doing a poor job. The brain's chemical messengers, also known as neurotransmitters, play a major role in all of these systems and networks, so let's take a closer look at them and how ADHD might be affecting them.

Neurotransmitters: The Brain's Chemical Messengers

At the very core of ADHD are imbalances in neurotransmitters. What are they? Neurotransmitters are chemical messengers that transmit signals between neurons and other cells in the body. They play a crucial role in muscle movement, sensory perception, and thinking and cognition. In essence, neurotransmitters are essential for the proper functioning of the nervous system since they allow communication and coordination between different parts of the body. So, what happens when these messengers get lazy, lost in the mail, or overeager? Well, it's a little chaotic, and all the systems will struggle to function properly, which is exactly what happens in the ADHD mind.

Key Neurotransmitters in ADHD

While there are many neurotransmitters in your body, there are four types that are highly affected by ADHD: dopamine, norepinephrine, GABA, and glutamate. The table below provides a simplified explanation of their role in the brain and how ADHD impacts their function. Understanding these key neurotransmitters can help make sense of why certain ADHD symptoms occur and why specific treatments or strategies may be helpful.

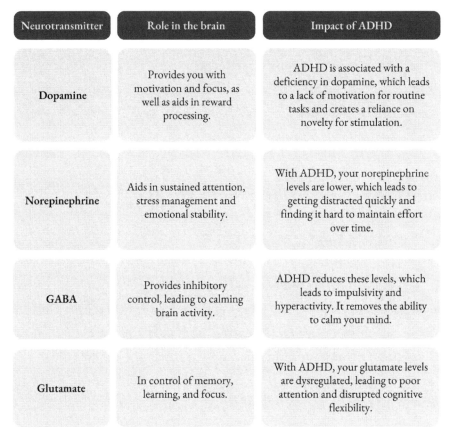

Neurotransmitter	Role in the brain	Impact of ADHD
Dopamine	Provides you with motivation and focus, as well as aids in reward processing.	ADHD is associated with a deficiency in dopamine, which leads to a lack of motivation for routine tasks and creates a reliance on novelty for stimulation.
Norepinephrine	Aids in sustained attention, stress management and emotional stability.	With ADHD, your norepinephrine levels are lower, which leads to getting distracted quickly and finding it hard to maintain effort over time.
GABA	Provides inhibitory control, leading to calming brain activity.	ADHD reduces these levels, which leads to impulsivity and hyperactivity. It removes the ability to calm your mind.
Glutamate	In control of memory, learning, and focus.	With ADHD, your glutamate levels are dysregulated, leading to poor attention and disrupted cognitive flexibility.

Table 2: Role of neurotransmitters and ADHD.

The Effect of Medication

The effects of ADHD on neurotransmitters are often treated with medication. While medication can't *cure* your ADHD, it can aid in the context of dopamine and norepinephrine. In this book, we'll look at strategies and tools to manage ADHD, but that doesn't mean that medication can't be helpful to you. For many people, ADHD medication has transformed their lives and allowed them to thrive in fields where they used to struggle. ADHD medications mostly target your dopamine and norepinephrine imbalances, aiding you to find a balance that will allow you to have improved focus, impulse control, and emotional regulation.

However, it's crucial to note that I am not a doctor, and this book isn't filled with medical advice. If you are considering using ADHD medications to help your neurotransmitters find balance, I highly recommend speaking to your healthcare provider about your options to determine what's best for you.

Why ADHD Feels Like a Tug of War

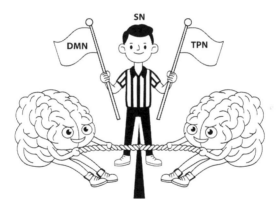

Okay, that was a lot of heavy information, right? So, let's take a little break by initiating our imaginations for a second. Take a moment to imagine a literal tug of war inside your brain. On the one side, we have the DMN, and on the other, we have TPN. Right in the middle, we have the SN acting as a referee. The DMN is trying to pull the TPN toward distraction and introspection, while the TPN is trying to pull the DMN toward focus and productivity. It's a continuous battle that can be quite exhausting and overwhelming at times. Unfortunately, this is a battle that the ADHD mind often loses because of two reasons:

- **The referee struggles to make a call:** More often than not, the SN struggles to switch modes, allowing one of the two competitors to break the rules. In most cases, it's the DMN that gets away with it, resulting in TPN losing the battle. However, sometimes, the referee switches sides and gets stuck on the TPN side. This leads to overexertion, like the crash you experience after intense hyperfocus.

- **Not enough fuel:** The TPN often loses the battle because it doesn't have enough fuel to keep going. What fuels the TPN? Mostly dopamine. When you are too low on dopamine, the TPN can't compete, allowing the DMN to win by default.

The result of this battle is a cycle of starting and stopping, zoning out, and struggling to stay consistent. It sounds pretty familiar, doesn't it? But more importantly, what can we do about this constant tug of war? The best thing you can do for your well-being is to reframe the tug of war.

Reframing the Tug of War

Reframing something means to change the way something is expressed or considered. It's like looking at a situation from a different angle or through a new lens. Reframing the tug of war means you're no longer seeing your ADHD as a villain. Your brain isn't broken. Is it different? Yes. Does it come with challenges? Absolutely! But is it all bad? Not at all. Instead of fighting the way your brain is different, let's welcome the different role-players and appreciate each other for what they bring to the table, starting with the DMN. Celebrate the DMN for being creative and reflective, and welcome TPN as your driving force to accomplish goals. When you no longer see one as the bad guy and don't resent your tug of war, you'll be able to learn how to manage the transition between the two phases better.

That's why understanding your brain is so important. It will allow you to notice which key players are in charge and make the most of each situation. In that way, you'll turn your tug of war into a balanced partnership.

ADHD Subtypes and Their Real-Life Impacts

The final part of fully understanding your ADHD lies in knowing the different subtypes of ADHD and their real-life impacts. Not everyone experiences ADHD in the same way. In fact, you can study two ADHDers and see very little similarities due to their different subtypes. While Attention Deficit Hyperactivity Disorder is the umbrella diagnosis, the subtypes can make a big difference in how you experience symptoms and which types of management techniques you need to focus on first. There are three subtypes of ADHD: inattentive, hyperactive-impulsive, and combined.

Inattentive

Inattentive ADHD, also known as Predominately Inattentive Presentation (PI), affects your ability to pay attention and focus. About 31% of adults with ADHD are classified as this subtype, and it can lead to individuals struggling to maintain focus on tasks, lectures, or even conversations (Wilens et al., 2009). With this subtype of ADHD, your mind will wander easily, causing a lot of issues with organizing and managing time. Inattentive ADHD is also characterized by forgetfulness and distractibility, as well as finding it really hard to remember details. If you find yourself daydreaming often, there is a good chance that you are an inattentive ADHDer.

If you have Inattentive ADHD, you might also experience symptoms of impulsivity and hyperactivity, and you might additionally struggle with impulse control and find it hard to keep your body still. However, these aren't the main symptoms of inattentive ADHD.

Inattentive ADHD is often overlooked in diagnosis because it's more internalized than outward. For example, children with ADHD are often characterized as kids who can't sit still or the ones who turn the classroom into a circus. However, a child with inattentive ADHD might be the *best-behaved* child in class. Don't be mistaken; they're not listening to a word you're saying. They're slaying dragons in their imagination. They're just not distracting everyone else as well, which means they're often over-looked.

Hyperactive-Impulsive

Hyperactive-impulsive ADHD is often the stereotype of ADHD. It's what every neurotypical imagines when you say you have ADHD. As the name suggests, it's characterized by impulsivity and hyperactivity. With this ADHD subtype, you are likely to fidget, squirm, and feel restless constant-ly. You might have difficulty sitting still and love to talk a lot. Additionally, you might also feel the need to touch and play with objects, even when it's inappropriate for the task at hand. For example, if you're visiting someone in the hospital, you might feel tempted to play with their chart or press the buttons that make the bed go up and down. Hyperactive-impulsive ADHDers are constantly on the go, and they tend to be very impatient. They might also act out of turn and forget to think about the consequences until much later. In adults, this might manifest as making inappropriate comments that seem funny in the moment, only to realize later it was hurtful.

Even though it's the most stereotypical archetype of ADHD, only seven percent of adults have this type of ADHD. In children, it's the most commonly diagnosed type since they are more likely to disrupt the classroom and cause chaos (Wilens et al., 2009). Typically, someone with this type of ADHD also finds it harder to manage emotions since they have the need to act on everything immediately without considering the future and consequences. It's not that they don't care about the future; they just struggle to consider it when emotions are running high.

Combined

Most adults experience a combination of inattentive and hyperactive-impulsive, which is known as combined ADHD. Combined means that you don't fall within just one of the other two categories but experience symptoms of both. ADHDers with combined types experience challenges with focusing and paying attention, as well as difficulties controlling their behavior and movements. When you have combined ADHD, it will impact all areas of life, including academic, social, and relationships.

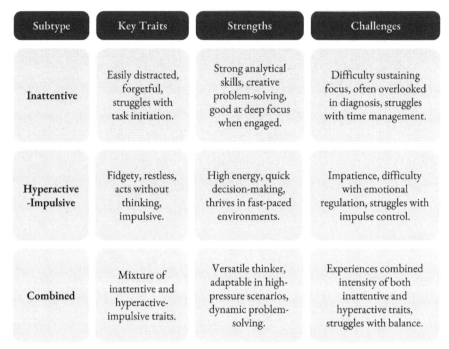

Subtype	Key Traits	Strengths	Challenges
Inattentive	Easily distracted, forgetful, struggles with task initiation.	Strong analytical skills, creative problem-solving, good at deep focus when engaged.	Difficulty sustaining focus, often overlooked in diagnosis, struggles with time management.
Hyperactive -Impulsive	Fidgety, restless, acts without thinking, impulsive.	High energy, quick decision-making, thrives in fast-paced environments.	Impatience, difficulty with emotional regulation, struggles with impulse control.
Combined	Mixture of inattentive and hyperactive-impulsive traits.	Versatile thinker, adaptable in high-pressure scenarios, dynamic problem-solving.	Experiences combined intensity of both inattentive and hyperactive traits, struggles with balance.

Table 3: ADHD subtypes and their key traits, strengths, and challenges.

Now that you have a clear picture of each type of ADHD, you'll have a better understanding of yourself, which will ultimately help you to implement and adapt different techniques so they can work for you effectively.

Chapter Takeaway

- Understanding the ADHD mind is important for implementing techniques that will work for you.

- The default mode network is the mind wanderer, distracting you with thoughts and providing reflection.

- The task-positive network is the doer who gets things done.

- The salience network serves as the switchboard operator, navigating between the DMN and the TPN. In the ADHD mind, this isn't always balanced.

- The limbic system is the emotional amplifier, and it can lead to emotional dysregulation due to unbalanced neurotransmitters.

- Neurotransmitters are the chemical messengers in your mind, and they all have different tasks. In ADHD, these messengers can be unbalanced, leading to ADHD symptoms.

- The unbalance can create a tug of war, but you don't have to resent the tug of war.

- There are different types of ADHD, including inattentive, hyperactive-impulsive, and combined.

Chapter 2

Why Traditional Solutions Keep Failing

"Strength does not come from winning. Your struggles develop your strengths. When you go through hardships and decide not to surrender, that is strength."

Gandhi

In Chapter One, we spent a lot of time learning more about the ADHD mind so we can understand what's really going on up there. When you understand your mind and the way ADHD is different from neurotypical minds, something special happens—a lightbulb moment where you realize why you've been struggling so much in life. Understanding the ADHD mind builds a strong foundation for the next step on the journey: realizing that you're not the problem. All those previous solutions you've tried that didn't work aren't due to a lack of trying. There are many other reasons why traditional solutions or solutions presented by neurotypicals don't work, which is what we'll unpack in this chapter.

First, we need to explore why neurotypical tools fall short, and then we'll explore the emotional toll of repeated failure. It's crucial to acknowledge the impact of repeated failure so you can understand why it's vital to seek tools and techniques that set you up for success and not failure. We'll also have a look at why other books marketed to an ADHD audience often fall short and why this book is different. So, make yourself comfortable and let's take a look at all our past failures. Fun!

Why Neurotypical Tools Fall Short

Studies have found that the ADHD brain thrives on flexibility and visual systems (Yin et al., 2022). Do you know what most neurotypical tools *don't* include? Flexibility and visual systems. No wonder they haven't been working for us! Most neurotypical tools are created in a linear way because (surprise) that's how a neurotypical mind functions best. It makes sense that they believe these types of tools are the best things since sliced bread because, for them, it is! But an ADHD mind, like yours and mine, works a little differently. Here are five reasons why neurotypical tools such as rigid planners and linear schedules don't work for ADHDers.

- **Executive function challenges:** The ADHD brain often struggles with executive functions such as planning, organizing, and time management. Turns out, you're not just a bad friend for forgetting about that coffee date with your friends; it's your brain! Because of the executive functioning challenges most ADHDers experience, the pressure to stick to rigid schedules and linear tools leads to a lot of frustration and feelings of overwhelm.

- **Difficulty with time perception:** ADHDers aren't great with time estimation. This is what we call time blindness. In other words, you struggle to understand how long tasks will take, which makes sticking to a rigid schedule unrealistic. Most ADHDers assume they can fit three days of work into one and then feel defeated when they can't achieve it, and linear schedules only add to the failure.

- **Hyperfocus:** Neurotypical tools don't take hyperfocus into account. When you become hyperfocused on a task, you might lose track of time and other commitments. A rigid schedule might disrupt the hyperfocus, causing an intense crash instead of riding the wave of productivity in that specific area.

- **Lack of motivation:** Rigid schedules are boring. I've never looked at an intense schedule and thought, *Wow, I can't wait to jump in.* Why not? Because there's no reward at the end of it. Here's a mind-blowing fact: Neurotypicals can accomplish tasks simply because they have to. Yup, they don't need additional motivation like most ADHDers, so their systems aren't created to motivate and reward. In other words, their tools don't have what we need to function.

- **Sensory overload:** Have you ever looked at a visual planner and thought, *What on earth are all these columns for?* There are so many traditional planners and tools that have features that I have no idea how to use (or why anyone would want to). A budget plan right next to my to-do list? Unless you want me to become distracted with my finances instead of focusing on the first task on my list, it's a no from me! Traditional planners have loads of *cool features* that might work for neurotypicals, but let's face it, ADHDers are going to have one look and feel overwhelmed (or totally forget about it after day two).

In Chapter One, we looked at the science behind why our brains work differently from neurotypical brains, but now we get to see it in action. Perhaps now you understand why your desk planner sounded like a good idea but ended up being a place to scribble down doodles or meeting notes. It wasn't created with your ADHD needs in mind. Let's be clear: Most neurotypicals don't provide poor advice and recommendations on purpose. They honestly believe that your ADHD will be managed by another day planner the size of an infant. The difference is that now you know and understand why it's not the best idea. These tools and tips aren't provided just to see you fail, but even good intentions can lead to failure. All those failed attempts at becoming the most organized person in your home or *getting it together* aren't because you're a failure. The tools failed you, and you might not even realize the emotional impact that's been having on your life.

Emotional Toll of Repeated Failure

I was recently visited by a very good friend of mine and her three-year-old daughter. My friend lives in the city, so she visits me often for a brief escape from the hustle and bustle since I live in a more secluded area surrounded by nature. Being in nature is always a treat for her little girl as well, as she doesn't often get the opportunity to look at wildlife and not cars and people. In anticipation of their visit, I purchased a small bug-catching net for my friend's little girl with the hopes that it would encourage her to play outside. As my friend and I were enjoying our coffees and chats, little Penny was running around with her net, just as I anticipated. What I didn't anticipate were the tears that followed soon after.

"Mama, I'm not good at catching bugs! I can't do it!" she cried. "Keep trying, darling," her mother encouraged her, continuing to sip her coffee. A few moments later, Penny cried again, "I'll never be able to do it! I'm not good enough." I felt awful. The tool I thought would keep her entertained was causing her turmoil. Her mother calmly called her over, wiped her tears, and then asked her to show us how she was using the net. Penny jumped into action, tucking the net side into her hand, running around with the wrong end sticking into the air, trying to slam the bugs out of the air. Recognizing our mistake in not showing Penny how to use the net, we couldn't help but laugh.

The Wrong Tools

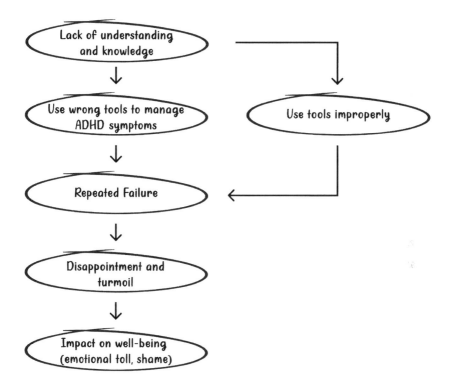

What happens when you use the wrong tools?

This encounter made me think of all the tools I've used in my life as an ADHDer and how much turmoil it has brought me. I realized again that day that I was never the problem. Often, the problem is we hand ADHDers tools to help manage their symptoms, but we don't explain how to use them. So, we end up using it wrong, which leads to more disappointment and turmoil than any good. Similarly, we're often given the wrong tools.

It's like running a marathon in flip-flops! You're not the problem, but the tool is wrong for you and your ADHD mind. Unfortunately, we usually don't realize it as quickly as in Penny's example. ADHDers spend years trying to use the tools they've been given, failing over and over again. And just like Penny, we feel like we're not good enough or like we'll never be able to accomplish anything.

Repeated failure can have a massive impact on your well-being and take a considerable emotional toll. When you're constantly trying to do things that others can do seemingly easily, but you're experiencing constant failure, it's bound to lead to shame. Shame is not the same as guilt. You might not feel guilty about missing another deadline, but you're sure to feel shame. *Shame* means "to hide or cover up" (Dodson, 2022). In other words, it's that awful feeling of wanting to hide that you've failed or hide yourself from others completely. I remember that feeling all too well! If I had a dollar for every time I hid my crumbled-up homework or permission slips so my friends wouldn't be seen, I'd be on a cruise ship right now.

Why Does This Matter?

Why is it important to be aware of this emotional turmoil? Firstly, so you can cut yourself a break and know that you're not alone. Repeat this after me: I'm not the problem. That doesn't mean we should go around blaming everything else. Instead, it should provide you with some comfort. You failed again? That's okay. That means it's time to make adjustments to the tools you're currently using. Secondly, it's important to understand this emotional turmoil so you'll feel encouraged to make the changes required. I know you might be used to failing by now and think that it doesn't affect you mentally and emotionally, but it does. You might not be feeling shame anymore, but perhaps you're feeling frustrated and angry. Or, perhaps past failure has placed pressure on you to always be perfect so you won't ever feel shame again. Regardless, repeated failure will affect you deeply, which is why it's time to let go of tools and techniques that aren't leading to success and embrace the tools offered in this book instead.

The Impact on Your Executive Function

The emotional impact of continuous failure can also greatly impact your executive function. Executive function is a set of cognitive processes that help with self-regulation, allowing you to effectively plan, prioritize, and sustain effort (*ADHD, Executive Functioning, and Shame*, 2023). Executive function is basically what allows you to make the shift from wanting to get things done to actually getting things done. However, in the ADHD mind, executive function difficulties are normal, which leads to time blindness, struggles with reaching goals, and difficulty with emotional regulation. Because of this, ADHDers tend to feel even more shame, which then makes executive functioning even less productive. It creates a nasty cycle just because your mind works differently.

Chances are, you've been called lazy or undisciplined before due to your difficulties with executive functioning. Being misunderstood only intensifies the fear of being a failure, and it usually leads to additional pressure to be perfect. That's why it's so crucial to surround yourself with people who understand you and your ADHD mind. But before you can expect someone else to understand, you need to understand it yourself. The best gift you can ever give yourself is some grace. In other words, understand how your mind is different and take that into account when you feel like you've failed at something. Instead of adding to your own emotional turmoil, choose to focus on tools and tips that will make you feel strong and empowered.

Why Other ADHD Books Often Miss the Mark

Have you ever found a new management tool or technique that immediately clicks? You're motivated to use this new tool, and you're more productive than ever. You even catch a glimpse of hope, thinking this is the start of something new—a life free from ADHD struggles. Then, a week or two passes, and suddenly, that exact same tool no longer works. What happened? Did the tool change overnight? Are you being dramatic? Did you lie to yourself about it ever working? When this happens, it can very quickly lead to a downward spiral of frustration and disappointment. If you can relate to this feeling, you're not alone. Most of the people I've worked with and helped have experienced the same disappointment in their lives, and it can really feel like a punch in the gut. So, what happened? Why did the tool or technique stop working? Probably the same reason why most other ADHD books miss the mark: it's too generic.

Most ADHD books offer a one-size-fits-all solution, completely failing to acknowledge the diversity within ADHD. While there are some tools that can absolutely be beneficial for all three subtypes of ADHD, most tools require some personalization or a completely different approach to applying them. For example, if you want an ADHD adult to function in a busy office, you'll need different approaches and tools. To help the hyperactive-impulsive ADHDers manage their energy and get their legs moving, the manager might ask them to run errands or work in collaborative groups. That way, they'll be moving their body and have a physical task to complete, helping them manage their ADHD and be less disruptive. However, if you ask the inattentive ADHDer to do the same, they'll most likely start dreaming about the pictures on their co-worker's computer screen and fail to listen to what the rest of the team is saying completely.

Now, please note that this is just an example, and it won't be the same for every inattentive or hyperactive-impulsive ADHDer. But that's kind of the point: even ADHDers with the same type of ADHD will respond differently to the same tools, and that's something most ADHD books don't recognize. For a tool to be effective, it needs to be adaptable and flexible. More specifically, the goal of the tool needs to be clear. If someone tells you to use a traditional calendar, what is the real goal behind it? Do you want to track progress or remember important dates? While neurotypicals might use one tool to achieve both goals, as an ADHDer, you might want to explore different tools to achieve different goals. Understanding what you want to achieve from using the tool will allow you to look for ways to adjust and adapt (or choose a different tool altogether) so it can provide you with the outcome you're looking for.

The thing is, most books also fail to acknowledge that a tool might work for only a period of time. While neurotypicals might use the same organization tool for the rest of their lives because it works for them, ADHDers are more likely to switch up their tools. What works for you today might not have the same results tomorrow, and that's totally okay. You don't need to hold on to a tool that no longer serves you. In other words, don't be married to one specific tool. If it's not working anymore, you need to be honest with yourself and begin to adjust and adapt to it.

Top Five Useless ADHD Tips and Tools

I'm sure you've received your fair share of useless advice over the years, and while it can be frustrating, I can't help but laugh most of the time. It used to upset me, but by understanding my brain, I've learned to accept it for what it is: useless. So, to show you that you're not alone, I would love to share my top five useless ADHD tips.

1. **Organizational binders:** No. Just no. No matter how much I've tried to use an organization binder, it always ends up as a collection of scrap papers, forgotten invoices, and random papers I didn't want to lie around on my desk anymore. Sometimes, I'll even shove the clean paper that doesn't fit into the printer into the binder. Out of sight, out of mind. Honestly, just get a trash can and recycle the papers. We all know you're not really going to go back and check what you put in the binder anyway.

2. **To-do list:** To-do lists can be helpful, but more often than not, they're more overwhelming than useful. Neurotypicals might look at a to-do list and feel motivated, but for many ADHDers, a to-do list seems impossible to complete, so why even get started in the first place, right? However, to-do lists can be helpful when used in the right way. It shouldn't be used to keep track of tasks or important dates. Instead, it can be used as a momentum builder to spend one hour being super productive. For example, if you need to clean your house, write down all the tasks and see how many you can tick in an hour.

3. **Phone calendars:** Similarly to to-do lists, they're not 100% useless. The problem is that most phone calendars require a multi-step process. For the calendar to be effective, you need to remember to look at the calendar each day. You also have to set alarms for the important tasks and dates you're entering into the calendar. In other words, you're likely to forget a step and then forget to check the calendar anyway. I find calendars useful for visually tracking progress or for birthdays and anniversaries, not for keeping track of work tasks. However, what doesn't work for me might still work for you.

4. **Try harder:** When someone says, "Just try harder," they com-

pletely ignore the neurological basis of ADHD. This piece of advice is about as useful as a bread knife that can't cut bread. The best thing to do with advice like this? Ignore it and know that you're already trying your hardest. Just because Uncle Steve doesn't realize it doesn't mean you're doing something wrong. Perhaps he should try to "Just be smarter."

5. **Notebooks:** Let me take a guess—somewhere in your house is a drawer or storage container with a plethora of nearly empty notebooks: Notebooks you wanted to use to write down due dates or to-do lists but ended up forgetting about them. Am I close? Most ADHDers want to be good at admin and want to keep track of things in a notebook. But that means you need to remember to use the notebook and look inside it. Most of the time, using notebooks only adds pressure and frustration and isn't helpful at all.

We've all received our fair share of useless advice, just like these, but what matters is what you do with it. You don't have to try to make other people's useless advice work. There are enough brilliant, helpful, and positive tools and tips that you can incorporate that actually work. So, see these useless tips for what they are and choose to focus on the ones that carry some value. By seeking value in tools and tips, you'll be able to create your own methods, schedules, and tools that work for you. Even if it works for literally no one else but is helpful to you, it's a success!

We can now take all that we've learned in this chapter and begin to apply it by evaluating the tools we are currently using. Are they really working for *you*? Or are you trying to make something work that wasn't created for your brain? In the next chapter, we'll look at some tools and tips that work (and those that won't) when it comes to emotional regulation.

Chapter Takeaway

- Neurotypical tools don't work because they are rigid and linear, while the ADHD mind thrives on flexibility and visual aids that aren't overwhelming (or cause sensory overload).

- Even though you're not a failure, you might be feeling like one due to all the failed attempts at using neurotypical tools and techniques.

- Repeated failure can have a huge impact on your well-being and a negative impact on your executive functioning, creating a cycle of repeated failure and losing confidence and hope.

- Other ADHD books on the market tend to fall short and miss the mark because they fail to incorporate adaptability and personalization. Generic advice won't work because every ADHD mind is different.

- It's okay to laugh every now and then at the awful tips you've received from other people and books claiming to hold all the answers; as long as you remember that their poor advice doesn't reflect on your abilities.

Chapter 3

Mastering Emotional Regulation

"This is the challenge of emotional self-control—having the appropriate emotion and feeling it at the right intensity. When it comes to getting things done, people with ADHD struggle with both sides of the equation."

Ari Tuckman

E veryone experiences emotions. Whether you're neurotypical or neurodivergent, you will, at some point in your life, experience emotions and be faced with a decision: How will I respond? Emotional regulation is the process of dealing with the emotions you're experiencing. In other words, it's your mind's way of processing and choosing how to respond and react to the emotions you're feeling. However, there are many players at work in the mind when it comes to emotional regulation. As the quote at the beginning of this chapter suggests, emotional regulation or self-control requires two steps: having the appropriate emotions and the right intensity. Unfortunately, both of those steps are things ADHDers tend to find challenging.

I remember when I was in high school, I would get into these really bad arguments with my friends and family. I would always burst into tears and storm off, feeling misunderstood and mistreated. It would feel so incredibly unfair and unwarranted that I was often tempted to throw a pillow across the room or swear never to speak to them again. I thought it was normal to feel that way. It's just a teenager being a teenager, right? Well, while teenage hormonal changes certainly didn't help, they weren't quite the cause. After all, every teenager experiences hormonal changes, yet it seemed worse for me than for most others.

As I got older, it didn't quite go away, which is when I realized it might have more to do with my ADHD and less to do with being a teen. It took me a long time and countless trials and errors to find techniques and tools for emotional regulation that actually work for me, and I would love to share them with you. In this chapter, we'll explore why emotional dysregulation is core to ADHD and why it's crucial to understand it. We'll then look at some quick-win strategies to deal with intense emotions and some advice on which tools to use and when. However, it's not just about short-term relief, so we'll also look at some techniques to help with building long-term resilience.

Are you ready to remove the emotionally loaded gun and regain control over your emotions? If not, that's also okay. Remember, you're not alone, and if you feel overwhelmed, take a five-minute break and then come back. This is your journey, and you can go as quickly or slowly as you want to.

Why Emotional Dysregulation Is Core to ADHD

Most people assume that emotional outbursts or intense emotions end after teenage years, but that's not entirely accurate. We still experience the same emotions, perhaps even more intensely, but we have better regulation systems. Or at least, the neurotypical mind is supposed to. The ADHD mind, on the other hand—not so much. Studies have found that ADHD adults are more likely to experience emotional outbursts of anger, impatience, and frustration. In fact, a study conducted in 2005 found that 32% of adults with ADHD showed serious issues with emotional dysregulation (Shaw et al., 2014). So, what does all of this mean?

It means that there's a reason you've been struggling with emotions your entire life. No, you're not just being *overdramatic* or *attention-seeking*, as you might have thought or been told in the past. There are scientific reasons as to why this is something you're struggling with. In fact, let's pause right here to look at some of the reasons why ADHDers tend to experience emotional dysregulation.

Lack of Norepinephrine

Has your day ever been ruined by a simple "k" text message? You and me both. There are very few things that can make me spiral like a cryptic text message. *What do you mean by "k?" Are you mad at me? Have you been in an accident and can only manage to type one letter? Are you absolutely deranged and assuming a "k" won't send me into a spiral, or are you doing it on purpose?* These kinds of thoughts can keep my mind occupied for hours. Well, not really, because I'll definitely overthink and escalate the situation by either calling you or blocking you because I'll assume our friendship has ended. Well, turns out I'm not being a *psycho* when this happens. It's actually due to a lack of norepinephrine.

We briefly chatted about this chemical messenger in Chapter One, but here's a quick recap. Norepinephrine helps the brain regulate responses to stress and maintain emotional stability. So, when the norepinephrine levels in your body are out of balance, you will experience a heightened sensitivity to stress. This also leads to struggles with calming down after an emotional trigger, which is why you might tend to harbor icky feelings toward others. For ADHDers, this is a daily struggle since norepinephrine levels aren't balanced within the ADHD mind, contributing to emotional dysregulation.

Feeling Overwhelmed

Due to the imbalance of chemical messengers in the brain, ADHDers are more likely to get stressed and overwhelmed by small things. The fact that most ADHDers have been told they are "lazy" or "careless" all their lives also contributes to feeling overwhelmed when the tiniest things go wrong. Let me explain.

I was told by many teachers and adults (and even peers) that I was careless and spoiled because I didn't take care of my possessions. I often lost brand-new shoes, misplaced toys, or forgot to put things away after using them. So, when I moved into my first apartment and couldn't find my keys, I freaked out. At that moment, I believed that they were all correct about me. I thought I *was* careless and spoiled because how could I possibly lose my only set of keys to my new apartment? I started freaking out and cried uncontrollably over the missing keys, and my poor boyfriend at the time had no idea what to do. "It's just keys," he tried, sending me into an even worse spiral. "You don't understand!" I yelled at him. Skip ahead a few hours, and you will find my boyfriend and I having the worst argument of our entire relationship, all because of a set of keys.

In my brain, it was never just about keys. The keys were simply the trigger for a much more emotionally loaded situation, and when he didn't understand, all the emotions started rolling out. And with no way to regulate those emotions, it turned into a big, relationship-ending argument. Unregulated emotions can greatly impact your relationship's health, as well as your work performance (Stange, 2021). That's why it's crucial to find solutions that work for you to successfully regulate your emotions.

I cannot stress this enough, but managing emotions is a cornerstone of thriving with ADHD as it breaks the cycle of shame and impulsive reactions. Emotional control won't stop you from losing your keys, but it will provide you with a choice: Do I want to lean into the chaos and lose my cool along with the keys, or do I want to take a step back, control what I'm feeling, and choose to react in a way that I won't be ashamed of later? In other words, learning how to manage your emotions is, in my opinion, more important than learning how to use a label maker so your office won't be as disorganized.

The Trial and Error Approach

Before we look at the actual tools and techniques that will be helpful in managing emotions, we need to have an honest conversation. The truth is your first attempt at regulating your emotions might not work. I'm not saying none of your attempts will work, but you need to embrace a sort of trial-and-error approach. You currently have no idea how your mind will respond to these tools and techniques, so you'll have to get to know yourself in the context of what works for you and what doesn't. The more times a tool or technique doesn't work, the closer you are to fine-tuning your techniques and finding one that is successful. The key lies in making each technique as personal as possible. If you don't relate to something, change it. Make it your own, and you will eventually find the right techniques.

I remember when I first tried emotional regulation strategies on myself. Some days, deep breathing worked like magic; other days, it felt like trying to stop a hurricane with a paper fan. I learned that switching things up—like adding a short walk or even a silly dance—kept me engaged and helped me find what worked in that moment. Flexibility is everything when it comes to ADHD, so don't limit yourself by adopting pressure for the first technique and tool to work. Remember, the goal isn't to find one fantastic and perfect tool that you can rely on for the rest of your life. The goal is to build an arsenal of tools to help you through various ups and downs. So, as we look at these quick wins for emotional control, remember to view these as your starting point, not as steps that are set in stone. Everything is customizable, even if that means combining three methods and creating your own little monstrosity of a tool. If it works for you, it's perfect.

Quick Wins for Emotional Control

Let's say for a moment you're in a packed elevator. There's a baby crying, an old man's phone is ringing, and he doesn't seem to notice, and the man behind you keeps pushing his shopping cart against your back. To make matters worse, you're already running late because your quick stop at the mall before the party took much longer than you anticipated, and you still need to get changed because you spilled coffee on your brand-new shirt. Oh, and did I mention you still need to wrap the gift you bought your friend? Emotions are running high as you feel completely overwhelmed and overstimulated. What do you do?

This might seem like a nightmare situation to most people, but I'm sure some neurotypical would say something like, "Well, if you planned better, this wouldn't have happened." Well, guess what, Susan, our brains don't work like that. You didn't choose to be in that situation on purpose, and to assume you could've simply done anything to avoid it is quite conde-scending and inaccurate. So, instead of thinking of what we could've done to prevent the situation (adding to shame), let's focus on quick techniques we can lean on to overcome the emotions in the moment.

Deep Breathing

Have you ever watched a movie where someone is freaking out, and then some other person tells them to "just breathe?" Most people assume this kind of advice is as useless as telling someone to "just calm down," but that's not actually true. Taking a couple of deep breaths can be incredibly beneficial to calm down your nervous system, allowing you to see things clearly and take control of your emotions. However, practicing deep breathing isn't always easy, especially when your emotions are already running at a thousand miles per hour. More importantly, when your emotions are triggered, most ADHDers won't even remember that deep breathing is an option. But if you try it once or twice and experience relief, you'll begin to automatically think of deep breathing when you are feeling overwhelmed.

So, why does it work? When your fight-or-flight response is on fire (like in a crowded elevator), your breath will automatically become more shallow. When you counter shallow breathing with intentionally deep breaths, it slows down the nervous system, allowing you to *relax*. By increasing your oxygen intake, more oxygen will reach your brain, allowing you to think clearly and reduce brain fog (Harris, 2020). To use deep breathing as a quick-win method, you can follow these easy steps.

- Close your eyes and begin to focus on your breath. Feel it as it enters through your nose and exits through your mouth. Focus on the temperature you're feeling as the cold air enters and warm air exists.

- Inhale slowly as you count to four and hold it for another few counts before you exhale slowly. Focus on nothing other than breathing and counting.

- Continue the pattern until you feel your heart rate calm down and your emotions simmer down.

Deep breathing might feel strange at first, but the more you do it, the easier it will become to regulate your emotions through breathing. Best of all, you can do it literally anywhere, and you don't need anything other than your breath and the ability to count. This is a great tool for when you feel overwhelmed; however, the intensity of your emotions is still fairly low.

Quick Distraction

Another great technique for when the intensity of your emotions is still pretty low is making use of quick distraction. Quick distractions are when you actively shift your focus onto something else so you no longer focus on the thing causing you overwhelming feelings. In other words, instead of cycling through all the things causing you sensory overload in the crowded elevator, you will choose to focus on something else that will distract you from what's overwhelming you. This works very well with the ADHD mind since it can quickly jump from one focus to another. By using this as a quick win, you're using what many people see as an ADHD weakness to your advantage to regulate emotions.

In other words, quick distractions work because you are interrupting the cycle of negative thoughts and feelings that can spiral out of control. There aren't exact steps to using quick distractions because something that might work for me might not work for you. However, here are a few examples of quick distractions that you can try:

- Make use of a fidget toy and focus on the sensation you're feeling as you touch the toy.

- Play music or put your headphones on. You don't have to listen to *calming* music. Instead, play a song that always puts you in a good mood.

- Play a memory game by naming as many animals as you can or by creating a poem where every sentence starts with the next letter of the alphabet.

- Take out your phone and look at old memories, or play a game (Candy Crush is still my go-to!).

- Switch your attention by doing something else with your body. For example, a few jumping jacks or a dance party (this might not work in the example of the crowded elevator, but I'll leave that decision up to you).

A quick distraction is a great way to quickly pull you out of the spiral of your emotions. Did it solve the issue? Of course not. But it helped you not to have a full-on panic attack or outburst, which is a win in my books!

5-4-3-2-1 Grounding Technique

If you're experiencing medium-intensity emotions, you might need something more powerful than deep breathing or a quick distraction. One of my favorite quick-win techniques for emotional regulation is the 5-4-3-2-1 grounding technique. Grounding exercises might seem too simple to work, but don't let the simplicity fool you. These types of techniques can be very effective as they allow you to bring yourself into the present moment and let go of intense emotions. It's also a technique that's very easy to use, and all you need is your senses.

The 5-4-3-2-1 grounding technique works because it removes the loaded gun (heightened emotions). It helps you to get out of the spiral and back into the present moment. In other words, instead of wanting to scream back at the crying baby, you'll realize that it might not be the best idea. Being in the present moment will provide you with clarity to respond to your emotions in a way that you won't regret later in the day. Here's how you can make use of the 5-4-3-2-1 grounding technique.

- **Sight:** First, you need to focus on five things you can see. It can be anything from patterns and colors to random objects in the room. For example, in a crowded elevator, you might see a blue hat, the green elevator button, the baby's red cheeks, someone's forgotten water bottle, and a suspicious stain on the floor.

- **Touch:** Next, focus on four things you can touch or feel. This can include the scratchy label inside your shirt, the hard floor underneath your feet, the ridges of your cell phone cover, and the cold touch of the metal handlebar you're holding onto.

- **Sound:** Begin to pay attention to everything you can hear. Focus on three specific sounds. This can include sounds that are overwhelming you since it won't do any good to put additional pressure on yourself not to hear them. Instead, see it as part of your game. You might be hearing the baby crying, the old man's phone ringing, and the *ping* of the elevator door.

- **Smell:** This is my least favorite part of the grounding, and for that reason, it always makes me laugh. Focus on two things you can smell. Perhaps it's the strong cologne of the teen boy who just walked in, or perhaps you've found the reason why the baby is crying; regardless, try to identify two smells.

- **Taste:** This might be tricky, but try to find one thing you can taste. Do you still have an aftertaste of your morning coffee? Perhaps you're eating a breath mint and can taste the freshness. Focus on one taste, even if it's the leftover garlic from your lunch.

You don't have to wait until your emotions are heightened to use the grounding technique. Many people do this grounding exercise daily to improve overall clarity and mental well-being. However, it's one of the best tools to rely on when you are in desperate need of quick emotional regulation.

Stepping Outside

The stepping outside technique is a simple yet very effective way to regulate emotions, especially for ADHDers. It involves taking a few moments to step away from the situation that's causing you to be stressed or overwhelmed and engage in a brief physical activity. This could be as simple as taking a quick walk, doing jumping jacks, or stepping outside for a few minutes to breathe in some fresh air. Why is this helpful? Because physical activity releases endorphins, which have mood-boosting effects. Physical activity also clears your head, providing you with a new perspective on things. Once you've calmed down, you can return to the situation with a clearer mind and better ability to cope.

In the case of a crowded elevator, if your emotions are heightened and you are feeling incredibly overwhelmed, you can physically step out of the elevator when it reaches the next floor. Even if you still have three more floors to go, get off immediately and use the stairs instead. As you're using the stairs, you will release endorphins, get your body moving, and allow your mind a moment to let go of the chaos it experienced within the elevator. In the same way, if you're in a heated argument and you feel your emotions are getting too intense, ask for an intermission and go for a walk or a quick workout. This will allow you to discuss the issues more clearly and calmly once you return.

This technique is very beneficial because

- it's quick and easy.

- it can be done anywhere.

- it's effective in reducing stress and anxiety.

- it will help you think more clearly.

- it will improve your mood.

Cold-Water Splash

Another wonderful quick-win method to use if you are feeling overwhelmed and your emotions are very intense is a cold-water splash. The cold-water splash technique is exactly what it sounds like. You literally stop what you're doing and splash cold water on your face. This can be done by filling a sink or bowl with cold water and cupping your hands to splash water onto your face. Another way to incorporate this is by using a spray bottle filled with cold water. Why is it helpful to splash yourself with cold water? The cold water stimulates the vagus nerve, which is responsible for functions such as heart rate, blood pressure, and digestion. When it's stimulated, it helps the body and mind to calm down (*Vagus Nerve Stimulation*, n.d.).

This technique is so easy and simple, yet incredibly effective. It's especially helpful if your emotions tend to lead to a lot of anxiety and stress. However, it can also be used to calm down anger and aggressive outbursts. I personally also use this technique when I'm struggling to concentrate or feeling *trapped* in my mind. Even if you have doubts about these techniques, try them and adapt them slightly so they work better for you.

However, remember that these are all quick-win techniques. You also need to invest in building long-term resilience.

Building Long-Term Resilience

While quick win techniques are helpful, you also need to think long-term. I know that's not most ADHDers' strong suit but bear with me. I'm not saying plan the next 10 years ahead of time. Instead, I'm asking you to invest in your future by taking care of yourself one day at a time. There are many techniques you can incorporate into your life that will help you build long-term resilience and improve your overall emotional regulation in the long run, including therapy, mindfulness, and celebrating every small victory. Let's take a closer look at each to see that it's not as intimidating as it might sound.

Therapy

Therapy can be daunting. What do you mean I have to tell a stranger all my darkest secrets? Well, that's not exactly what therapy entails. In fact, most therapists don't care that you, at the age of seven, fed your sister's Barbie doll to the dog on purpose because you were jealous. Therapy isn't what most of us imagine it. Therapy can be a very powerful tool for building long-term resilience and improving emotional regulation because it can help you identify and understand your triggers. In other words, instead of waiting for your emotions to get triggered, you can begin to understand why they were triggered in the first place. By pinpointing specific triggers, you can develop proactive strategies to manage the emotions before they escalate.

Therapy is also useful because it allows you to develop healthy coping mechanisms. While therapy isn't a quick fix and more of a journey, it allows you to build skills and tools that will last. However, therapy is collaborative, and you need to find a therapist who not only understands ADHD but understands *your* ADHD. Don't feel pressure to commit to the first therapist you visit. Instead, do some research, set up some meetings, and choose a therapist you feel most comfortable with.

Mindfulness

Mindfulness is another powerful tool for building long-term resilience and regulating emotions—but before you roll your eyes at yet another mindfulness suggestion, hear me out.

I get it—sitting still, focusing on your breath, and "clearing your mind" sounds like an absolute nightmare for the ADHD brain. And if you've ever tried traditional mindfulness only to find yourself three minutes deep into a mental monologue about what you forgot at the grocery store, you're not alone.

But mindfulness isn't about emptying your mind—it's about learning to guide your attention back when it wanders, without judgment. For ADHDers, this skill is life-changing. Instead of getting hijacked by intrusive thoughts or emotional overwhelm, mindfulness helps you press pause, break the cycle of negative thought loops, and regain control over your focus and emotions.

And the best part? You don't have to sit cross-legged in silence for an hour to make it work. Here are ADHD-friendly ways to make mindfulness *actually doable and effective* in your daily life.

- **Body scan**: A traditional body scan asks you to mentally "scan" your body from head to toe, noticing tension and releasing it as you go. Sounds good in theory, right? But in reality, it can take too long, and before you know it, your mind is off planning next week's schedule. **ADHD-Friendly Hack**: Instead of scanning your whole body at once, break it into micro-moments. Focus on *just one* body part at a time (hands, shoulders, jaw). Use a "tense and release" technique—clench your fists, then relax them. Do the same with other body parts.

- **Tactile objects:** One of the biggest ADHD challenges is getting stuck in your head—whether it's overthinking, spiraling into self-doubt, or getting lost in an imaginary debate from two years ago. The quickest way to break that loop? Engage your senses. **ADHD-Friendly Tactile Mindfulness**: Hold a textured object (a smooth rock, a piece of velvet, a fidget toy) and really focus on how it feels. Try temperature awareness—run cold water over your hands, sip a hot drink, or hold an ice cube. Experiment with scents—essential oils, a scented candle, or even something nostalgic (freshly ground coffee, anyone?).

- Mindful Movement: Good news—mindfulness doesn't require stillness. In fact, ADHD brains often benefit from mindful movement, which allows you to channel your energy while staying present. **ADHD-Friendly Movement Ideas:** Tai Chi (slow, intentional movements that sync with your breath), yoga (a mix of movement, balance, and deep breathing plus, a great excuse to stretch, dancing (freestyle or structured, it engages multiple senses at once), walking meditation (instead of sitting, try walking slowly and focusing on each step, how the ground feels, and the rhythm of your breath).

Celebrating Small Wins

I love celebrations. I'm not one of those people who *forget* when it's their birthday and don't want a big deal. I want a big deal; thank you very much. In general, there are few things that inspire me as much as celebrating. Whether I'm celebrating myself or others, it makes me happy and removes tension or negative emotions. That's why celebrating small wins is a great way for ADHDers to ensure that they don't just focus on all their failures but celebrate the progress they've made as well.

Celebrating small wins involves actively recognizing and appreciating even minor achievements. It could be completing a small task, overcoming a distraction, or simply showing up for oneself. These celebrations can take various forms, from a simple mental pat on the back to a small reward or sharing the accomplishment with a supportive person. The key is to make the celebration meaningful and personalized. You can shift your focus to progress and build a stronger sense of self-efficacy by intentionally acknowledging and celebrating small successes. Celebrating small wins doesn't have to be elaborate. Here are some practical ideas that can easily be incorporated into your daily routine:

- **Quick recharge:** Take a five-minute break to listen to your favorite song, stretch, or simply close your eyes and breathe deeply.

- **Mindful snack:** Enjoy a piece of fruit, a square of dark chocolate, or a handful of nuts while savoring each bite.

- **Digital detox:** Step away from screens for 15 minutes and engage in a hobby you enjoy, like reading, drawing, or playing a musical instrument.

- **Gratitude practice:** Jot down a few things you're grateful for in a journal or share them with a loved one.

- **Physical activity boost:** Go for a short walk, do a few jumping jacks, or dance to an upbeat song.

As you can see, there are many ways to master emotional regulation, some might be a more long-term approach, while others are great for in-the-moment usage. As long as you work toward the sustainability of management techniques, you're moving in the right direction!

Choosing What Works for You

With all of these great tools and techniques for your availability, you might feel slightly overwhelmed with choices. Where does one even begin, knowing that it will also require further modification before it works? Well, before the carriage runs away with the horse, let's take a deep breath. These tools and techniques are here to help you, not to add stress and fear. And to my empath friend: no, the techniques you don't pick won't feel left out. All you have to do right now is ask yourself: what tool do I feel like trying? If you're not sure which techniques will work for you, that's totally okay. Instead of putting pressure on yourself to pick the *right* one, take a moment to ask yourself the following questions that will help you understand yourself better, as well as identify your emotional patterns.

- Think of a time when you felt overwhelmed by frustration. What triggered that feeling?

- How do you usually respond when you feel overwhelmed?

- Have you ever felt better after reacting to feeling overwhelmed? What was it that you did? (For example, a shower, eating a meal, calling a friend, playing computer games, etc.).

- When you look at all the strategies presented in this chapter, which one feels easiest to try right now, and why?

- What makes you eager to manage your emotions more effectively? What would managed emotions look like to you?

Once you've asked yourself these questions, use the answers to guide you in picking your first technique to try. If all else fails and you feel no closer to making a decision than you were before you asked yourself all the questions, pick one at random and let fate decide for you.

Preparing for Setbacks

As mentioned in the trial-and-error approach section, your emotional regulation tools and techniques are bound to fail sometimes. But what do we do when our tools fail? Do we throw out the baby with the bathwater, or do we take a second to assess what aspect of the tool didn't work? Hint: it's the second one. To help make the assessment a little easier, you should be prepared for setbacks along the way. Preparing yourself for setbacks doesn't mean assuming everything will fail all the time. Instead, it's creating a plan of action if something goes wrong and the method you've been using no longer helps.

I once had a client, Jake, who came to me frustrated after trying a grounding technique that worked for his friend but left him feeling more agitated. "How am I supposed to let energy flow through my body? What does that even mean?" he asked me frustratedly. We talked about how different brains respond to different tools and how his brain wanted clear instruction and not "mindful-speak." After our discussion, we determined that it would be better for him to de-escalate his emotions with a cold-water splash. After a few tries, he discovered it worked wonders for him. The takeaway? Just because something doesn't work the first time—or at all—doesn't mean you're failing. It just means your brain needs a different key.

Preparing for Emotional Setbacks

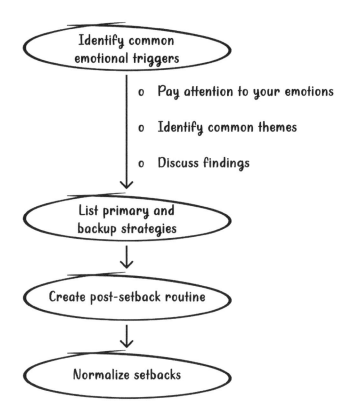

Instead of getting frustrated when something isn't working for you, let's follow these steps instead and create a simple plan for managing setbacks.

Identify Common Emotional Triggers

The first step in preparing for setbacks is becoming aware of what triggered your emotions. Identifying triggers can be a very powerful tool in taking care of your mental health, and it will allow you to understand yourself a bit better. Knowing what triggered you, you'll be able to draw patterns and find out why the chosen technique didn't work. It's not always an easy task to find what triggers you, but perhaps these simple steps will help you get to the root of your triggers.

- **Step 1—Pay attention to your emotions:** Start by becoming more aware of your emotions throughout the day. Notice when you feel happy, sad, angry, anxious, or any other strong emotion. Take note of the intensity and duration of these feelings. If you know you're going to forget, make a note on your phone and set a few reminders throughout the day to check in with yourself.

- **Step 2—Identify common themes:** Review your notes and look for recurring situations, people, or events that seem to trigger strong emotional responses. Think about your personality and what you usually experience more. Are you more prone to certain emotions, such as anger, anxiety, or sadness?

- **Step 3—Discuss findings:** You don't even have to discuss it with someone else. You can discuss it with yourself as long as you voice your findings out loud. Why? Because often, when we talk and hear ourselves, we finally process what's happening and receive additional clarity and revelation.

Once you've identified the common emotional triggers, you're ready for the next step in preparing for setbacks.

List Primary and Backup Strategies

We just discussed the process of choosing which strategies to use, but as we know, the ones we choose might not work out. When it comes to selecting tools and techniques to manage your emotions, it's best not to put all your eggs in one basket. Instead, choose one or two primary strategies, but have a backup. You can be fully invested in your chosen method and still have a backup in case they don't work out. For example, if you want to try a cold splash next time you feel overwhelmed, keep stepping out as a ready alternative if the cold splash doesn't work. Who knows, you might find that the alternative ends up working much better than the primary.

Create a Post-Setback Routine

Preparing for a setback means you need to be prepared for what happens immediately after. Do you tend to feel like a failure when you experience a setback? Do you tend to eat all your emotions away instead of dealing with them? Well, use that knowledge to your advantage by creating a simple post-setback routine for yourself. For example, I give myself ten minutes to feel all the emotions I want to within the safety of my room, office, or car. I put a timer on, and once the 10 minutes are finished, I stop myself in my tracks, drink a glass of ice-cold water, wash my face, and go for a walk. On the walk, I asked myself, *Why did that feel so extreme? What method did I try? Why didn't that method work? How can I adjust the method to work better for me next time?* Doing this stops me from relying on unhealthy coping mechanisms to avoid my emotions or facing the fact that it didn't work.

Normalize Setbacks

It's completely normal to experience setbacks on your ADHD journey, especially when it comes to managing emotions. I know it's easier said than done, but don't get discouraged if you have one bad day or feel like you're not making progress as fast as you want to. Everyone's journey is unique, and finding the methods that work for you will take some time. Allow yourself to feel your emotions, but resist the urge to give up. Even when you don't see progress, keep going. Celebrate the small victories, learn from your challenges, and be patient with yourself. There are many resources available to help you find the right tools for you, but you'll have to kiss a few frogs before finding your prince. Perhaps this next tool, the personalized solutions table, will help you to keep track of your progress and normalize setbacks.

Personalized Solutions Table

The personalized solutions table is a helpful tool that allows you to track your emotions, what triggered you, and the primary and backup strategy you tried. Most importantly, it encourages you to reflect on what worked and what didn't. Sometimes, there are elements of a specific strategy that work well, but a small portion that doesn't. Instead of dismissing the entire strategy, you can brainstorm ways to adjust and adapt it so all aspects of the strategy work for you. That's exactly what the personalized solutions table allows you to do. Here's an example of what it might look like.

Emotion	Trigger	Primary strategy	Backup strategy	Reflection
Frustration	Criticism at work that felt harsh.	5-4-3-2-1 Grounding.	Stepping out for fresh air.	Worked partially as I felt better. Next time, I'll try a walk instead of just stepping out.
Anxiety	Looming deadline.	Deep breathing.	A short walk and listening to some uplifting music.	Reduced anxiety, but I got distracted and wasted time. Next time, I'll use a timer for my strategies.
Overwhelm	Too many tasks to accomplish in one day.	Cold-water splash.	Quick distraction.	Felt much better after the cold-water splash, but the quick distraction led to procrastination. Next time, try using only the primary.

Table 4: Example of a personalized emotional regulation solutions table.

Creating a table for yourself will provide a way to keep track of the tools and techniques you've tried and the success you've experienced with each. This will also allow you to track your triggers, providing you with valuable information going forward.

You should view all these possible tools and strategies as apps on your phone. Sometimes, they need some customization before they're helpful. Other times, they simply need to be updated, and eventually, the app might get deleted if you no longer find it useful. Adapting these strategies is absolutely crucial, and it will greatly impact the success of your emotional management journey.

You won't get it right every time, and that's okay. The point isn't perfection; it's persistence. Keep showing up for yourself, keep trying, and keep adjusting. Over time, you'll find what works for you, and that's where real progress begins. Persistence is a common theme when it comes to treating ADHD symptoms, and it's one you'll continue to see in the next chapter as we look at how to create sustainable systems for productivity.

Chapter Takeaway

- Managing emotions can be very tricky, especially for ADHDers.

- Emotional dysregulation is at the core of ADHD due to a lack of chemical messenger and feeling overwhelmed.

- You can use quick-win methods for emotional control, such as deep breathing, quick distraction, grounding techniques, stepping outside, and a cold-water splash.

- Methods that contribute to long-term resilience include making use of therapy, implementing mindfulness practices, and celebrating small wins.

Chapter 4

Developing Sustainable Systems for Productivity

"Passion isn't everything, but everything is better with passion, especially if you have ADHD. I hope that you all find that passion about something or someone. Never stop looking for it. Once you find it, fight for it with every breath."

Shayne Neal

When my sister was little, she struggled heavily in school. I didn't admit it back then, but I liked that she also struggled. It showed me that, at least, if there was something wrong with me, I wasn't alone. We were in it together. I know it sounds cruel, but in my little mind, I found peace in our struggles because we had one another. However, one day, my sister came home from school with a letter from her teacher, sharing with my parents that she believed my sister needed glasses. Desperate for some answers, my parents took both of us to the optometrist, and a couple of hours later, my sister had glasses, and I had a lollipop and a high-five for having perfect eyesight.

After the initial adjustment to the glasses, my sister's life was transformed. Her grades improved, she actually enjoyed studying, and she even took up painting. Turns out, if you can see flowers for the first time and not just be aware of blobs all around you, you feel pretty inspired to capture them. While I was glad for my sister, I was also sad because, once again, I was alone with my struggles. Briefly after that, I got diagnosed with ADHD, and I was so excited to have my "glasses" moment, but it never came. There was no *tool* the doctors gave me that suddenly opened my eyes to a whole new world. It was just me and my struggles who now had a name.

If only I knew back then what I know now, that there are tools that can help. It might not be as immediate as glasses, but with time and adjustment, it can transform your life. In this chapter, we'll look at a few tools and techniques for productivity that are specially designed to help the ADHD mind. So, if you're desperate to have your "glasses" moment, this is it. But let's first start by looking at what makes a system ADHD-friendly.

What Makes a System ADHD-Friendly?

An ADHD-friendly system is one that is designed to accommodate the unique challenges and strengths of ADHDers. But what makes an ADHD-friendly system *actually* ADHD-friendly? There are five elements that every ADHD-friendly system needs.

- **Flexibility:** An ADHD-friendly system must be adaptable and able to change as your needs evolve. Life with ADHD is dynamic, with fluctuating energy levels, changing priorities, and unexpected challenges. A rigid system will quickly become frustrating and counterproductive. Instead, the system should be easily adjusted. This might involve modifying deadlines, changing the order of tasks, or incorporating new strategies as needed. Flexibility allows for individual preferences and accommodates unexpected circumstances, reducing stress and increasing motivation.

- **Simplicity:** Complexity is the enemy of ADHD. Overly complicated systems, with numerous rules and intricate procedures, can quickly become overwhelming and lead to avoidance. An ADHD-friendly system prioritizes clarity and ease of use. It should be intuitive and straightforward to understand and implement. This might involve minimizing the number of steps involved, using clear and concise instructions, and utilizing visual aids to enhance comprehension. Simplicity reduces cognitive load and makes it easier to stay on track.

- **Brevity:** Most ADHDers struggle with maintaining focus on long-term goals. One way to combat this is by breaking down larger tasks into smaller chunks. This can significantly improve motivation and reduce feelings of overwhelm. This approach, often referred to as *chunking*, allows you to experience a sense of accomplishment more frequently. The system reinforces positive behavior and encourages continued effort by celebrating small victories along the way. Brevity also makes it easier to adjust the system and adapt to changing circumstances without feeling overwhelmed by the prospect of a complete overhaul.

- **Rewards and incentives:** Positive reinforcement is crucial for maintaining motivation and encouraging sustained effort. An ADHD-friendly system should incorporate a system of rewards and incentives to celebrate accomplishments and acknowledge progress. These rewards can be intrinsic, such as a sense of pride and accomplishment, or extrinsic, such as a small treat, extra free time, or a desired activity. The key is to choose rewards that are meaningful and motivating for you. By recognizing and celebrating successes, the system fosters a positive feedback loop that encourages continued engagement and reinforces desired behaviors.

- **Accommodation for distractibility:** Distractibility is a hallmark of ADHD, and any effective system must address this challenge. This may involve creating a dedicated workspace free from distractions, utilizing noise-canceling headphones, or employing techniques like the Pomodoro Technique to break down work into focused intervals. Technology can also be a valuable ally in managing distractions, with apps and software available to block distracting websites, filter notifications, and track time spent on tasks. By proactively addressing potential distractions, the system helps you stay on track and minimize the impact of these challenges on your productivity and well-being.

In contrast, systems that aren't ADHD-friendly will have elements that are rigid, complex, and focus on punishment instead of reward. Furthermore, a non-friendly system will also disregard distractibility, lack visual cues, and focus mostly on long-term goals. Examples of systems that aren't ADHD-friendly include traditional educational systems, most workplaces, and even household routines. No wonder most ADHDers feel *blind* for their whole lives... but no more! Let's look at some tools and techniques that are ADHD-friendly and good for productivity.

Tools and Techniques That Work

To create a system that works for you, you need tools and techniques that fit into the system. Think of your system as your very own toolbox. Inside the toolbox are all kinds of tools (and techniques) you can rely on. Some days, you might need a hammer—something that's more structured, like time blocking. On other days, you might need a screwdriver—a more relaxed system that will allow you to plan your week like a to-do list. The goal is to fill your toolbox with the right tools and then use the right tool for the job. You can't hammer your way through every situation (like a rigid routine). You need to be prepared to swap tools every now and again.

Finding tools and techniques to put into your ADHD toolbox can often feel like online shopping—except the color filter is turned off, so you only see everything in black and white. It's a guessing game, and when your package arrives, you're surprised that you ever thought you'd like the bright orange sweater. It can be tricky, especially when so many techniques and tools are marketed as "ADHD-friendly," even when it's not. So, let me remove some of the guessing for you and present four tools and techniques that actually work for the ADHD mind. The best part of it all? You can further adjust and change each of these tools and techniques to better fit your needs.

Kanban Board

If you have no idea what a Kanban board is, don't worry! In short, it's a visual project management tool that helps you organize and track tasks. It typically consists of three columns: "To Do," "Ongoing," and "Done." Each task you have to do is represented by cards or sticky notes that are moved across the board as they are completed. You can also use it digitally if you prefer. There are several apps with this functionality. I use this type of board daily, and it's so satisfying to move cards around.

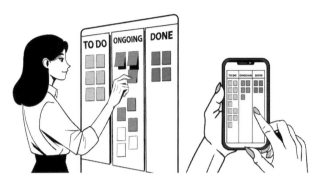

Kanban boards are considered ADHD-friendly for several reasons. First, they provide a visual representation of tasks, which can be helpful for ADHDers who may have difficulty with abstract thinking or organization. Second, they allow you to break down large tasks into smaller, more manageable steps, which can be less overwhelming and more motivating. Third, they promote a sense of progress and accomplishment as tasks are moved from one column to the next.

Kanban boards are not only ADHD-friendly, but they also help ADHDers be more productive in a number of ways. First, they can help you stay organized and focused by providing a clear visual representation of their tasks. Second, they can help you prioritize tasks and avoid feeling overwhelmed by the sheer number of things you need to do. Third, they can help you track your progress and celebrate your accomplishments, which can boost motivation and self-esteem.

One of my clients, Michelle, is an ADHDer with two ADHD kids. Keeping track of her own deadlines and her children's became an impossible task. Between making sure all her work was done, the house was clean, dinner was prepared on time, and her children did all their homework and chores, she needed something visible to remind her of all the tasks at hand. I suggested she try using a family kanban board. The family kanban board contained all the chores, all the due dates, and all the special occasions. It kept track of chores and tasks and even prompted when it was time for a fun surprise or reward. Setting up the board took some time and trial and error, but now she swears by it.

Pomodoro Timer

The Pomodoro Technique is a time management method that involves working in focused bursts followed by short breaks. It's named after the tomato-shaped kitchen timer used by its creator, Francesco Cirillo (*The Pomodoro Technique*, n.d.). To use this technique, set a timer for 25 minutes and work on a single task of your choice undistractedly. Once the time is up, you take a 5-minute break. After four subsequent pomodoros (25-minute work intervals), you take a break of 15-30 minute break.

This technique is considered ADHD-friendly because it aligns well with the attention spans of many ADHDers. The Pomodoro Technique helps combat feelings of overwhelm and procrastination by breaking down big tasks into manageable chunks. Additionally, the frequent breaks provide opportunities to recharge and prevent mental fatigue, which can be significant for any ADHD mind. Lastly, the visual and auditory cues of the timer can help maintain focus and provide a sense of structure and predictability.

The Pomodoro Technique can help minds like ours be more productive in several ways. First, it improves focus and concentration by providing a structured framework for work. You can better manage your attention and avoid getting sidetracked by eliminating distractions and setting a clear time limit. Second, it enhances time management skills by providing a tangible measure of progress. By tracking the number of pomodoros completed, you can gain a better understanding of how long tasks actually take and make more accurate time estimates in the future. Finally, frequent breaks can help to reduce stress and anxiety, which can be significant obstacles to productivity for ADHDers. By incorporating regular breaks into their workflow, you can avoid burnout and maintain a more sustainable pace of work.

Todoist

I know I mentioned earlier that some apps just don't work for the ADHD mind. A lot of apps require more effort to set up than it is helpful, and most of the time, ADHDers forget about the app after a week. However, some apps can be game changers, like the popular to-do list app Todoist. Todoist is a task management app, and it's considered ADHD-friendly because it is flexible, simple, and visual (Josel, 2024). There aren't any over-complicated features or anything that requires too much effort, making it perfect for the general ADHDer.

One of my favorite features of the Todoist app (not sponsored, by the way) is the way it breaks down large tasks into smaller, more manageable sub-tasks. It uses the chunking technique to make overwhelming projects feel less daunting and more achievable. Todosit also allows users to prioritize certain tasks and set due dates with automatic reminders, which aids in time management and combating forgetfulness.

Todoist also offers a variety of customization. Your app can look exactly how you want it to look, and if you get tired of it after a couple of weeks, you can switch it up! In other words, Todoist can enhance productivity by providing a framework for organizing thoughts and tasks while also providing freedom of flexibility and customization. By visually representing to-do lists and tracking progress, the app can help you stay on track, reduce feelings of overwhelm, and experience a sense of accomplishment as you complete tasks. Additionally, the ability to access tasks across multiple devices ensures that important information is always readily available, minimizing the risk of forgetting crucial commitments (Josel, 2024). So, if you forgot your phone at home but have your laptop with you, it won't feel like the end of the world.

Pascal, a client of mine, loves starting her day by creating a to-do list, but physical to-do lists often make her feel overwhelmed. Well, that was if she remembered to look at the to-do list during the day and not misplace it somewhere in her office. So, she switched to a digital to-do list, like Todoist. Instead of getting overwhelmed, she felt encouraged. With every big task broken up into more manageable tasks, she felt a surge of energy as she could complete so many tasks in one day (instead of just one big thing). The auto-reminders also helped her to constantly keep herself on track and not get sidetracked by other, more exciting things.

Eisenhower Matrix

The Eisenhower Matrix, also known as the Urgent-Important Matrix, is a time management and prioritization tool that actually works and categorizes tasks into four quadrants based on their significance and urgency. This method was popularized by former U.S. President Dwight D. Eisenhower, who famously said, "I have two kinds of problems, the urgent and the important. The urgent are not important, and the important are never urgent" (Team Asana, 2024).

The Einsenhower Matrix

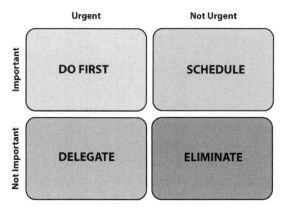

The four quadrants of the Eisenhower Matrix are:

- **Do First:** These are both important and urgent tasks. They must be immediately tackled. Examples include pressing deadlines, important meetings, and crises.

- **Schedule:** These are tasks that are important but not urgent. They should be scheduled for a later time when you have more time and focus. Examples include long-term goals, planning, and relationship building.

- **Delegate:** These are tasks that are urgent but not important. They can be delegated to someone else or, if possible, eliminated altogether. Examples include emails, phone calls, and interruptions.

- **Eliminate:** These are tasks that are neither urgent nor important. They should be eliminated or avoided altogether. Examples include time-wasters like excessive social media use, watching TV, or playing video games.

The Eisenhower is an ADHD-friendly method because it helps ADHDers prioritize their tasks in a way that makes sense. Instead of simply saying, "prioritize," it shows the user how to prioritize. It's also effective in breaking down large tasks into smaller, more manageable ones, improving productivity and reducing the chances of feeling overwhelmed. You can also further customize the Eisenhower to fit your specific needs by using visuals to represent the four different quadrants, by using a timer so prioritizing doesn't take the whole morning, and by being flexible in moving tasks from quadrant to quadrant.

ADHD-Tailored Planners

The last ADHD tool I want to present to you is not just one specific tool but rather a type of tool. While traditional planners often end up gathering dust somewhere (because you can't remember where you put it down, nor do you remember that you need it), an ADHD-tailored planner can add a lot of focus and organization to your life. So, what's the difference? ADHD-tailored planners are designed to cater to the unique organizational challenges faced by ADHDers. These planners incorporate features that address distractibility, difficulty with time management, and the tendency to become overwhelmed by large tasks (*ADHD Planners & Tools for Organization*, 2023). In fact, I created an ADHD-friendly planner with these principles in mind, which I introduced at the beginning of the book, you can go and download it anytime.

Naturally, the key feature of an ADHD-tailored planner is flexibility. Without flexibility, it's not ADHD-friendly, no matter what the marketing says. ADHD-tailored planners utilize visual aids such as color coding, mind maps, and checklists. The visual approach helps ADHDers see what they have lined up for their day instead of reading what they have to do. By minimizing complexity and maximizing visual appeal, these planners can reduce the cognitive load and make planning more accessible and enjoyable.

Furthermore, ADHD-tailored planners also emphasize positive reinforcement and reward systems. They may include spaces for tracking progress, celebrating accomplishments, and acknowledging successes. This focus on positive reinforcement is highly motivating for ADHDers, especially those who struggle with maintaining motivation and experiencing a sense of accomplishment. These planners can foster a sense of self-efficacy and encourage continued effort by recognizing and celebrating your achievements. In other words, ADHD-tailored planners provide you with what your mind needs to be productive and organized. Will you transform into Mary Kondo and become the most organized person alive? Nope. But will you remember to do the simple task you've been putting off for weeks? Yes, you will!

Creating Your Systems

Now that you have various tools available, you might be wondering: Where do I even begin? Well, there's good news and bad news. The good news is that you *get* to choose where you begin. The bad news is that you *have* to choose where to begin. If that thought makes you feel a little overwhelmed, that's okay. We'll figure this out together. All you need is a simple three-step plan: picking a tool, customizing it and then maintaining it.

Creating Your Systems

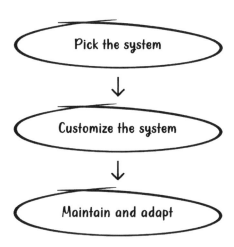

Picking the System

Picking the *right* system means picking a system that you feel drawn to. However, there are some guidelines as to which methods are more likely to work for you. Here's a little cheat sheet you can use to point you in the right direction:

- If you are a visual learner or generally more drawn to visual methods, start with a Kanban board or a simple mind-mapping technique.

- If you struggle with attention or you're experiencing a short attention span on one day in particular, use time blocking or the Pomodoro technique.

- If you get easily distracted, I suggest using a white noise machine and having a dedicated workspace where there are no distractions.

Customizing the System

Once you've picked a system, it's time for the customization to begin. You can chop and change whatever you want as long as it promotes productivity and organization for you. Remember, you're not creating a system that works for everyone or the majority of people. You're creating one for you. So, make it your own. To help you identify areas of customization, ask yourself these questions:

- What time of day do you feel most alert and focused? (Morning bird, night owl, or something in between?)

- Do you work better in short bursts or longer stretches? (Experiment with the Pomodoro Technique or other time-boxing methods.)

- What are your biggest time-wasters? (Social media, email, excessive web browsing?)

- Do you procrastinate more on certain types of tasks? (Creative projects, tedious chores, etc.)

- How do you best learn new information? (Visual aids, auditory explanations, hands-on activities?)

- Do you find it easier to remember information when you write it down, type it, or record it?

- How do you prefer to store and access information? (Physical notebooks, digital files, cloud storage?)

- Do you prefer visual or written planning methods? (Mind maps, to-do lists, calendars?)

- Do you find physical or digital tools more helpful? (Bullet journal, planner app, whiteboards?)

- What level of detail is most helpful for you in your planning? (Broad outlines or detailed schedules?)

- Do you find it easier to stick to plans that are rigid or flexible?

- What motivates you to stay organized? (Rewards, sense of accomplishment, reducing stress?)

- How can you reward yourself for completing tasks? (Small treats, breaks, leisure activities?)

- What are your biggest obstacles to staying organized? (Lack of motivation, distractions, feeling overwhelmed?)

- How can you make your chosen system more enjoyable and engaging? (Personalize it with colors, stickers, or your favorite themes.)

- How can you adjust your system as your needs and priorities change? (Regularly review and revise your methods.)

- What support systems can help you stay organized? (Accountability partners, family members, therapists?)

Now that you've explored different ways to customize your system, it's time to take a step back and track what actually works for you. The diagram below serves as a visual aid to help you choose the right tools based on what you're trying to accomplish. The goal is to make it easier to get started and reduce some of the overwhelm.

Customizing Your Systems

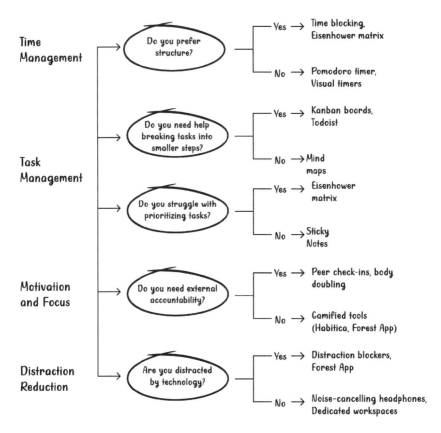

Now that you have some viable options for tools and techniques that really work, it's time to face the next challenge when it comes to productivity and organization: keeping track of the tools you've tried and figuring out what works for you and what doesn't. That's why this next tool is an absolute game-changer!

Personalized Productivity Planner

A personalized productivity planner is a table for goal-oriented experimentation with tools, tracking what worked and what didn't, as well as possible alternatives you can make in the future. This personalized productivity planner will help you keep track of your progress, and it will allow you to constantly assess whether strategies and tools are working for you. It will allow you to get to know yourself even better as you begin to recognize patterns of which goals work best with which tools. Here's an example of what a personalized productivity planner might look like.

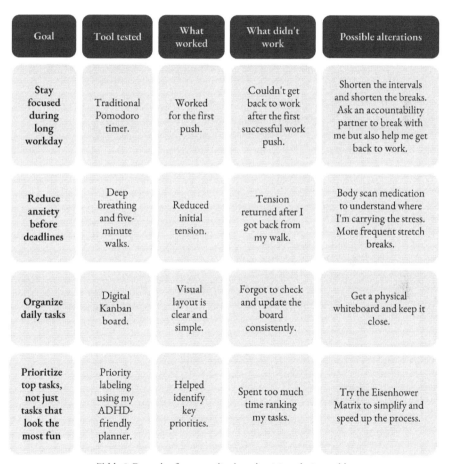

Goal	Tool tested	What worked	What didn't work	Possible alterations
Stay focused during long workday	Traditional Pomodoro timer.	Worked for the first push.	Couldn't get back to work after the first successful work push.	Shorten the intervals and shorten the breaks. Ask an accountability partner to break with me but also help me get back to work.
Reduce anxiety before deadlines	Deep breathing and five-minute walks.	Reduced initial tension.	Tension returned after I got back from my walk.	Body scan medication to understand where I'm carrying the stress. More frequent stretch breaks.
Organize daily tasks	Digital Kanban board.	Visual layout is clear and simple.	Forgot to check and update the board consistently.	Get a physical whiteboard and keep it close.
Prioritize top tasks, not just tasks that look the most fun	Priority labeling using my ADHD-friendly planner.	Helped identify key priorities.	Spent too much time ranking my tasks.	Try the Eisenhower Matrix to simplify and speed up the process.

Table 5: Example of a personalized productivity solutions table.

This is an example of how you can use this productivity planner and keep track of what works for you and what doesn't. Remember, there's no shame if your first approach doesn't work. Keep going, and eventually, you'll find a system that works for you.

Maintaining and Adapting Systems

We've all been there: You have the sudden urge to clean your office space. So, you put on your comfy pants, grab a few trash bags, and begin throwing the contents of every drawer onto a pile in the middle of the floor. After multiple energy drinks, a few breakdowns, and long hours, it's complete. Your office looks spectacular! The pens are color-coordinated in the drawer, your files are labeled and filled with the corresponding papers, and your office plants have been watered for the first time in months. You feel on top of the world, and you promise yourself that you'll keep everything as it is. How hard can it be, right? Well, skip forward a couple of weeks, and the chaos is back. Why? Is it because you didn't care enough? Or is it because the systems you have in place don't work? Actually, neither of those answers is necessarily correct.

Sometimes, even the systems that work can fail. How? Because we have the right productivity and organization systems, but we don't have the right tools to maintain and adapt these systems. To help in this area, here are two things that will help you maintain and adapt your systems.

Accountability

Accountability is a vital component of maintaining ADHD-friendly systems because it provides external motivation. This helps you to overcome the inherent challenges of procrastination and difficulty with follow-through. By sharing your goals and progress with others, you can increase your commitment to your systems and receive support and encouragement from your loved ones. You can receive accountability in various ways, and two of the most helpful ways include body-doubling and check-ins.

Body Doubling

Body doubling is a technique that involves working alongside another person while you complete a task. The other person doesn't need to provide guidance or feedback; their mere presence acts as a powerful motivator. Knowing that someone else is witnessing your efforts can significantly increase focus and reduce distractions. This method is particularly effective for tasks that require sustained attention, such as studying, writing, or completing chores. For example, let's say your system to keep your room clean is to sort out the pile of clothes on your chair every Friday evening. However, this one particular Friday evening, you really don't feel up to it. But how would you feel if your partner was sitting on the bed, keeping you company while you sorted your clothes? Chances are, it now sounds like a much better time. Here's why body doubling is beneficial.

- **Increased focus and motivation:** The presence of another person can help you stay on task and resist distractions.

- **Reduced procrastination:** Knowing that someone is observing you can make it harder to procrastinate.

- **Improved time management:** Body doubling can help you stay on track and complete tasks within the allotted time.

- **Enhanced social connection:** Working alongside another person can provide a sense of camaraderie and support.

Peer Check-Ins

Peer check-ins involve regularly sharing your progress and challenges with a trusted friend, family member, or accountability partner. This can be done through regular meetings, phone calls, text messages, or online platforms.

During these check-ins, you can discuss your goals, track your progress, identify obstacles, and brainstorm solutions. Check-ins don't have to be formal, but they need to be intentional. In other words, have your accountability buddy check in once a week to ask you about your progress. Now, I know this sounds annoying or like you're being babysat, but more often than not, having someone checking feels caring and heartwarming when it happens at the moment. Just imagine having a friend checking in after a super busy week, and you get to share and celebrate with them all the things you've accomplished. Or, if you had a bad week, you'll have someone who listens and offers advice and encouragement for the following week! Here's why check-ins are so beneficial:

- **Increased motivation and commitment:** Sharing your goals with someone else can increase your commitment to achieving them.

- **Improved problem-solving:** Discussing challenges with a trusted partner can help you identify solutions and develop effective strategies.

- **Enhanced support and encouragement:** Receiving support and encouragement from a peer can boost your motivation and help you stay on track.

- **Reduced feelings of isolation:** Connecting with others who share similar challenges can reduce feelings of isolation and increase your sense of belonging.

External Motivators and Rewards

Accountability is the first piece of the puzzle when maintaining and adapting your systems. The second piece is finding external motivators and rewards. External motivators and rewards play a crucial role in maintaining your systems. We know that ADHD often presents challenges with intrinsic motivation, making it difficult to find the internal drive to complete tasks that may seem tedious or unfulfilling. That's why external motivators, such as praise from others, recognition for achievements, or tangible rewards, can provide the extra push you need to stay on track and maintain momentum.

These rewards can be tailored to your individual preferences and can range from small treats and breaks to larger rewards like special outings or new gadgets. You can increase your engagement, improve your persistence, and experience a greater sense of accomplishment by incorporating external motivators and rewards into your systems. However, even with accountability and external motivators, there is a possibility that your systems will stop working. What happens then? Well, in the wise words of Ross Geller from the sitcom *Friends*, that's when we "Pivot!"

When Systems Stop Working

Sometimes, systems stop working. They don't give a one-week warning sign or provide a visual representation of how effectively they are still working. One day, they work, and the next, they don't. There's no shame in that. The trick lies in knowing when to keep going because you're simply having a bad day or when to ditch the systems and start over. Let's be honest: Most ADHDers, when they feel overwhelmed, begin to toss things in the trash. While sometimes that's necessary, it's not always the right move when it comes to systems. However, to know when it's time to start fresh, we first need to know why the system stopped working in the first place.

Why They Stop Working

Let me start by saying that it's totally normal for systems to stop working. Life with ADHD is dynamic, and there are many struggles that fluctuate. One week, you might be in constant hyperfocus and need reminders of when to go to the bathroom, while in other weeks, you can't think for more than two minutes at a time. So, naturally, the same systems won't always work. Here are three reasons why systems stop working for you without warning.

The Need for Novelty

ADHDers thrive on novelty and excitement. So, when a system begins to feel like a boring routine and becomes too predictable, your mind might begin to reject it as it loses its appeal. Instead, your brain will seek out new stimuli, leading to distractions and a decline in adherence to the system. To prevent this from happening, you can introduce new elements or variations to the system to keep it engaging and interesting. This could involve trying new techniques, experimenting with different approaches, or adding some fun to the system.

For example, I find it helpful to play soft music (without lyrics; otherwise, it ends up in a concert featuring me) while I'm doing a work push. However, I recently began to notice that music no longer helped me to get started and didn't keep me entertained anymore. Instead of scraping the system altogether, I went on eBay and bought a vintage record player. I still had a box of records that I inherited from my grandad, so I started using that as my source of music, adding some excitement back into my system.

Changing Circumstances

Life with ADHD is rarely static. When everything is changing, why do we expect our systems to continue working? While the ADHD mind likes novelty and change, it also struggles to adjust old routines to fit new places. For example, if you move to a new apartment, your old systems might suddenly not be as effective as they were in your old home. However, changes don't even have to be that extreme to warrant systems to stop working. Something as *minor* as changes in symptoms or responsibilities can trigger systems to stop working. In other words, these changes will require adjustments to the system to ensure it remains effective and supportive. Ignoring changes in your circumstances won't do any good, so it's better to acknowledge them and decide preemptively to adopt new approaches.

System Burnout

System burnout occurs when you become overwhelmed and exhausted by the constant effort required to maintain your systems. This can happen when the system itself is too rigid or demanding, leading to feelings of stress, frustration, and, ultimately, a sense of failure. When you experience burnout, you may feel drained, demotivated, and unable to sustain the effort required to follow your systems. This can lead to a sense of hopelessness and a feeling of being trapped in a cycle of failure.

It's important to recognize that system burnout is not a sign of weakness or a lack of effort. It is a natural consequence of the challenges associated with ADHD and the constant effort required to manage symptoms and navigate daily life. By acknowledging the possibility of burnout and taking steps to prevent and address it, you can maintain your systems and continue to make progress toward your goals. In rare cases, even well-designed,

ADHD-friendly systems can lead to system burnout. This occurs when you've been relying on one system for a long time, and your brain starts to view it as *boring*.

What Does This Mean for ADHD Minds?

When systems fail, it can feel like a personal failure. It can add a lot of pressure and guilt, which won't do you any good. Instead, embrace the idea of change. It's okay to switch things up when something isn't working. If you want to change something for no reason, it's probably your brain encouraging you to try something new and switch things up. So, don't reject those prompts. Experimenting with new systems can lead to improved self-awareness and understanding of your personal preferences. In other words, don't be scared of change. I know that's easier said than done, so here is some practical advice for switching things up and keeping your mind intrigued by the systems you have in place.

Practical Advice

When systems stop working, you might be met with an initial panic. What now? Should I start from scratch? Are all of my systems going to stop working now? I understand the panic, and it's okay to feel the emotions you're experiencing. However, before you spiral out of control, here are a few practical things to do to prevent this panic. In fact, these three practical steps should be done constantly, not only when you experience a system breakdown.

When Systems Stop Working

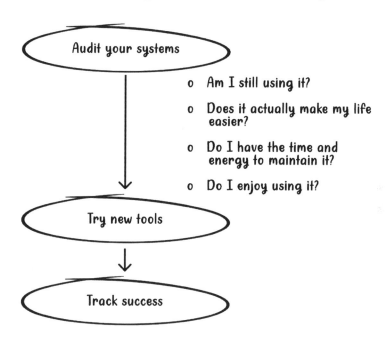

Audit Your Systems

Firstly, you need to audit all the tools and techniques you're using in your current system. Auditing your systems means assessing every element of your system. Ask yourself questions like, *Is this tool still serving me?* If the tool isn't working anymore, you'll start to see signs that will prompt you to try something new before the system shuts down completely. Here are a few other questions you can ask yourself as part of the audit.

- **Am I still using it?** This is a very important question because if you're not using it, it won't work, no matter how good the system is.

- **Does it actually make my life easier?** A lot of the time, tools sound like they'll make your life easier, but it ends up being more admin than anything else. Even if it's a tool you paid money for, don't cling to it just because you want it to work. If it doesn't make your life easier, it's time for a new one.

- **Do I have the time and energy to maintain it?** If a system requires too much upkeep, it's not sustainable in the long run. If you're spending more time crafting your calendar every day or updating your online task board than you're actually spending on your work, it's not a long-term solution. No ADHD technique should be that complicated to keep up to date.

- **Do I enjoy using it?** If you're dreading using your system, you're less likely to stick with it. It's important that your system brings you joy and provides you with the right dopamine boost to start your day. If you're not enjoying the system, it's time to switch it up.

Try New Tools

When you've audited your system, you'll know which tools need to be swapped with something else. Perhaps you can return to methods you've relied on in the past, but maybe it's time for a brand-new tool. Trying new tools might feel scary, but try to see it as unboxing a surprise box. You won't know how well it works or whether it was worth it until you open the box. Trying new tools is a great way to build resilience and not be freaked out when systems stop working.

One of my clients, Carla, used to be very reluctant to try new tools. She would know for weeks that her current system wasn't working anymore, but she was reluctant to change it. One day, she decided to start by making small changes. For example, she switched to an online calendar with auto-reminders instead of using a physical one. She noticed that the small changes made a big difference, and it helped her grow in her confidence. Now, she loves change, and she often switches up her systems to keep herself entertained and make everyday tasks seem more exciting.

Constantly trying new tools also removes the constant pressure to be perfect. Instead of worrying about a system that might fail, you can have the freedom to try new systems and fail miserably but learn from your failures.

Track Success

The last step is to track your success. The productivity planner is a great way to do this. That way, when a system fails and you need new tools to use, you can refer back to your productivity planner and assess what might work for you. You might notice that you tried a tool once and found it helpful but didn't make it part of your system, which you can now. Tracking your success also means focusing on how much you've gained, not just every time you feel like you failed. When a system begins to fail, instead of beating yourself up, take a moment to reflect back on all your successes and celebrate those instead. Let them inspire and encourage you to keep going, even when you don't want to.

The perfect system doesn't exist—but the perfect system for you? That's something we can create, tweak, and rebuild over time as long as you remain flexible and curious and continue building your toolbox. As we wrap up looking at techniques and tools to help with productivity, it's time to take a look into the future. What's next on this epic journey? Exploring the impact of ADHD on social situations and relationships.

Chapter Takeaway

- An ADHD-friendly system needs to be flexible, simplistic, brief, rewarding, and distraction-free.

- Tools and techniques that work for ADHD productivity include the Kanban board, Pomodoro timer, to-do list apps, Eisenhower Matrix, and ADHD-tailored planners.

- To create your system, you need to start by picking a system based on what you're naturally drawn to, and then you should customize it further to suit your needs and wants.

- The personalized productivity planner is a great way to conduct a goal-oriented experiment and keep track of all the tools and techniques you've tried.

- To maintain and adapt systems, you need to adopt a sense of accountability and use external motivators and rewards.

- Systems can stop working at any given time without any warning due to your brain's need for novelty, changing circumstances, and system burnout.

- When systems stop working, you need to audit your systems, try new tools, and track your success.

Chapter 5

Relationships and Social Dynamics

"One thing people with ADHD wish other people knew, is that we don't ignore, forget, and not listen on purpose. As much as it irritates, offends, and hurts you... it makes us feel just as embarrassed, guilty, and sad."

Unknown

When I met Biance, she had just gotten out of a two-year relationship. It was clear that the wounds were still pretty raw, and she often teared up when we spoke about it. She still loved her ex-partner very much, and she regretted the way things ended. "What do you think happened?" I asked her early on her journey, to which she shrugged and said, "It's the two-year curse." Turns out that every close relationship, whether romantic or not, never lasted beyond two years. We worked together to find management techniques for organization and emotional regulation; she eventually admitted that she was ready to discuss how ADHD can impact relationships. I knew it was an incredibly hard step for her to take, but I was excited about the breakthrough awaiting her.

We spent many hours discussing how ADHD, specifically her ADHD, has affected her relationship. We dug deep and assessed all the relationships she felt were affected by the *curse*. After much discussion and soul-searching, she realized that there was no curse—only her ADHD. While it was hard to face the truth, she had to realize it in order to implement the right tools to ensure stronger connections in the future. That's exactly the journey we'll be exploring in this chapter.

We'll start by looking at the various ways that ADHD can impact relationships. We often overlook this area of effect because we assume ADHD only impacts work and academics. However, many relationships are deeply affected by ADHD and emotional dysfunction. We'll then look at tools every ADHDer can implement for stronger connections, with a special focus on the flexibility and adaptability of these tools. It's vital to know that not every tool will work for you, and that's okay. Setbacks are normal, and it's how you respond to the setbacks that really matter. So, are you ready to dig a little deeper into your relationships and how your ADHD has impacted them? I know it might be uncomfortable, but it's not as uncomfortable as losing connections because of misunderstandings.

How ADHD Impacts Relationships

One of the biggest misconceptions about ADHD is that it only affects certain areas of our lives. The truth is that ADHD knows no boundaries. It doesn't bother you at work, and then it decides to leave you alone when you're with your spouse. ADHD isn't something that you can switch off, and therefore, it affects all areas of your life, including relationships. Struggles and conflict are normal in every relationship, but there are certain ADHD symptoms that add a little fuel to the fire, making it hard to work through issues without them interrupting into flames. Things like forgetting anniversaries, interrupting your partner when they're speaking, or zoning out as they're sharing their day with you can be quite frustrating for the non-ADHD partner. Does the ADHD partner do it on purpose?

Of course not. It's probably just as frustrating to the ADHDer, especially when they know they've unintentionally hurt someone they love.

Common ways that ADHD impacts relationships include

- **Communication breakdowns:** When you get easily distracted by internal thoughts or external stimuli, it makes it really hard to listen and respond appropriately to every conversation. Communication is also impacted by ADHD due to emotional outbursts and trouble explaining why they are feeling a certain way. This can lead to irritability and withdrawal.

- **Impulsivity:** ADHDers can sometimes act impulsively or make spur-of-the-moment decisions without fully considering the impact on their relationships. This can add a lot of pressure on the relationship. Initially, it might be fun and exciting, but it can quickly lead to stress and the ADHDer being unreliable in the context of the relationship.

- **Misunderstandings:** Due to challenges in understanding and considering other people's points of view, ADHD can lead to misinterpretations and miscommunications. Something might make perfect sense in your mind but not to your partner, and vice versa.

I often explain the impact of ADHD on relationships to my clients as a ripple effect.

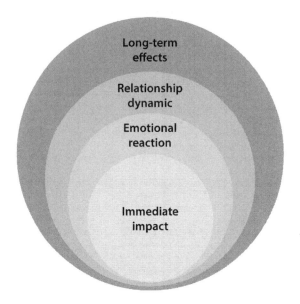

- **The first ripple—Immediate impact:** The first is the initial impact of the impulse that took place. For example, let's say you forgot an important date. The immediate impact might be confusion and minor annoyance from your partner.

- **The second ripple—Emotional reaction:** Based on the immediate impact, you and your partner will have an emotional reaction. Your partner might feel hurt and frustrated with your forgetfulness, while you might feel misunderstood.

- **The third ripple—Relationship dynamic:** Due to the emotional reaction, your relationship dynamic will change. Your partner might begin to trust you less and have growing resentment toward you, while you might internalize it and pull away.

- **The outer ripple—Long-term effects:** Due to the change in the dynamic, there will be lasting relationship change. This is where there is a need for active repair or, in severe cases, where breakups occur.

As you can see, a minor ADHD behavior can lead to a serious impact, especially when no relationship repair takes place. However, ADHD doesn't have to be the end of your relationship. With the right management tools and the support of a patient partner, you can make your relationships work. Trust me, for a very long time, I thought I'd never meet someone who'd understand my ADHD and love me for it. In past relationships, I often felt the need to pretend like I was perfect, but that only led to even more frustration and fear. Now, I'm happily married to a man who supports and loves me through all my ups and downs. Not only does he research ADHD so he can better understand me, but he also helps me implement tools and strategies to ensure our connection grows stronger over the years. Speaking of which, let's take a moment to explore some of the ADHD-friendly tools for stronger connections.

Tools for Stronger Connections

What does it mean to have a strong connection with someone? Does it mean you never disagree? Does it represent a relationship that's perfect without any problems? Not at all. Having a strong connection means having a deep and meaningful bond that goes beyond surface-level interactions. It's a sense of closeness, understanding, and trust that allows you to feel comfortable and safe when you're around them. In other words, as an ADHDer, strong connections provide you with a place to be yourself while also welcoming the other person to do the same. As much as you need acceptance, understanding, and patience, so do neurotypical people.

That means that these tools won't transform you and your relationship into some special Hallmark movie where everything is perfect. Instead, these tools will give you the ability and opportunity to go beyond the surface with your friends and romantic partners. These tools will help you to manage the ripples of ADHD in your relationship in a way that adds to your relationship, not increases the tension. Let's take a look at five tools you can incorporate to aid in stronger connections.

Active Listening

The first tool that can aid in fostering stronger connections is the art of active listening. Active listening is a communication technique that involves paying close attention to what someone is saying, both verbally and nonverbally. In other words, instead of just *hearing* someone, you're actually *listening* to someone. Have you ever found yourself knowing that someone spoke to you, but you can't remember a thing they said even though it happened three seconds ago? Well, that's because you're hearing and not listening—and me saying that is not trying to make you feel bad about yourself. I am very guilty of this myself. It took me many years and many tools to get to a place where I can listen to others without thinking of how I can add to the conversation.

As ADHDers, we often hear what someone is saying and want to make them feel like we understand. So, we interrupt them by sharing a similar story that we experienced ourselves. In our minds, it makes sense. We're saying, "Hey, I get how you're feeling because this happened to me, which made me feel a similar way." Unfortunately, that's not how it's perceived. What the other person is hearing is, "Oh, you don't actually care how I feel, so you're going to make it about yourself... again." This miscommunication can be hurtful to both parties, which is why active listening is crucial. Sometimes, people just want to be listened to. Active listening involves the following principles:

Active Listening

```
┌─────────────────────────┐
│     Pay full attention   │
└─────────────────────────┘
            ↓
┌─────────────────────────┐
│     Show engagement      │
└─────────────────────────┘
            ↓
┌─────────────────────────┐
│  Ask clarifying questions │
└─────────────────────────┘
```

- **Paying full attention:** Focus on the speaker, maintain eye contact, and avoid distractions like your phone or other thoughts

- **Showing you're engaged:** Use nonverbal cues like nodding, leaning in, and making appropriate facial expressions to show you're interested and engaged in the conversation.

- **Asking clarifying questions:** Ask open-ended questions to encourage the speaker to elaborate and ensure you understand their message fully. For example, instead of saying, "Ah, that sucks," you could ask, "How did that make you feel?"

The benefits of active listening are overwhelming, and it includes improved communication, stronger relationships, increased empathy and understanding, and conflict resolution. A client of mine, Pedro, struggled immensely with listening to instructions, stories, and conversations. As soon as his turn to speak was over, his mind would wander off and switch to something else (which often led to interrupting his partner). Since he started implementing active listening, he's been able to listen to his partner without interrupting her and actually pay attention to what she's saying (even the little details). Not only does it make him feel better, but it also improves their relationship since his partner now feels more appreciated and listened to. While active listening might not work for everyone, it's a wonderful technique to try if your partner is constantly making you aware of the fact that you appear like you're not listening to them.

Clear and Direct Language

Clear and direct language is another communication tool that can help improve relationships and cultivate stronger connections. It prioritizes straightforwardness and conciseness while it aims to convey information in a way that is easily understood. Clear and direct language means you have to be honest and transparent with the person you're in a relationship with. You can't expect to cultivate a deep connection with someone if you're not willing to be vulnerable. However, clear and direct language means you have to put aside your people-pleasing tendencies. Instead, you need to communicate clearly what you are experiencing. Key characteristics of clear and direct language include:

- **Simplicity:** Use simple and familiar words that are easy to understand. Avoid jargon, technical terms, or complex sentence structures.

- **Conciseness:** Get to the point quickly. Avoid unnecessary words, phrases, or details that don't add value to the message.

- **Specificity:** Be specific and concrete in your language. Avoid vague or ambiguous terms that could be interpreted in different ways.

- **Clarity:** Structure your message in a logical and organized way, making it easy to follow. Use clear transitions and signposts to guide the listener or reader.

- **Directness:** State your message directly and assertively. Avoid beating around the bush or using a passive voice.

Clear and direct language doesn't mean sharing everything you think or being rude. Instead, it means expressing how you're feeling and how you're experiencing certain things in a way that others can understand. For example, if you're feeling overwhelmed after a long and busy day at work and your partner comes home and immediately asks what's for dinner, clear and direct language won't mean lashing out. It also doesn't mean pretending like you're fine. Instead, it might look something like this: "Honey, as much as I want to share a meal with you tonight, I am exhausted. I experienced a lot of issues today, and it took all my energy to stay on track and make decisions. Would you please decide what's for dinner?"

Using clear and direct language will help you become a more effective communicator and improve your ability to connect with others.

Setting Reminders

How many times have you gotten into an argument or conflict with someone in your life because you forgot something? Whether it's signing permission slips, remembering dinner plans, or celebrating anniversaries, I've forgotten them all in the past. But let's be honest for a moment: In a world with so many ways to stay connected and be reminded, using "I just forgot" won't cut it anymore. While it's not your fault for struggling to remember things, it is your responsibility to ensure that you take note of the things that are important.

Setting reminders shows thoughtfulness and care. You can set them to remind you of important events, such as birthdays and school trips, or to remind you of smaller things, like checking in with your friend who's been going through a difficult time. Reminders can help you stay in touch with friends and loved ones, deepening the bond between you. Remember, reminders are just one tool in your relationship-building toolkit. They should be used in conjunction with other communication and relationship-building strategies, such as active listening, empathy, and showing genuine interest in others. Some of the best reminder apps include RescueTime, Freedome, Evernote, and Mint.

Clarifying Expectations

Clarifying expectations means ensuring that you and the person you're in a relationship with both understand what is expected of you. It means openly discussing with one another what you both expect from the relationship, even if it's a friendship. I almost lost a very close friend of mine due to unmet expectations. After she had her baby, I had assumed she'd want some space to be alone and settle in. What I didn't know was that all our other friends were going to visit her. Truth be told, I might have been invited to join and missed the email, but I was unaware of the meetup at the time. My absence really hurt my friend as it felt to her like I didn't care. I thought I was being thoughtful, while she felt like I was being selfish.

We can laugh about it now because neither of us expressed our expectations prior to the birth of her baby. If we only stopped to check in with one another, it would've prevented the whole ordeal. If I sent her a text with a simple, "Hey, in my mind, I believe you want space after you have the baby and won't want to see anyone. Is that accurate of me to assume, or would you like me to come over?" A simple text would've taken less than a minute to craft and saved hours of tears and animosity.

Clarifying expectations also enhances trust and intimacy in a romantic relationship. When you feel heard and understood, you are more likely to trust and open up to your partner, which can lead to deeper levels of intimacy and connection in your relationship. Unmet expectations can lead to stress, anxiety, and frustration for both partners. Clarifying expectations can reduce uncertainty and create a more predictable and comfortable environment for everyone involved.

Repeating Key Points

Repeating key points goes hand-in-hand with active listening. This tool can be of great value for building deeper connections with others because it can improve communication by providing clarity and focus. Repeating key points ensures that the message is understood correctly, reducing misunderstandings that can arise from distractions or difficulty processing information. For example, if someone is sharing something with you and you're unsure what you mean, you reflect it back to them as a question. Repeating key points also allows you to maintain focus on the conversation, especially when you're dealing with complex or emotional topics.

Repeating key points shows that you're actively listening and valuing what the other person is saying. It demonstrates empathy and understanding. You also create a shared understanding of the conversation, fostering a sense of connection and trust by repeating key points. This will reduce anxiety and stress in the relationship, and knowing that your thoughts and feelings are being heard and understood makes it easier to connect on a deeper level. You can practically use this tool by doing the following:

- **Summarize:** After the other person speaks, summarize the main points in your own words to ensure you understand correctly.

- **Ask clarifying questions:** If you're unsure about something, don't hesitate to ask clarifying questions to ensure you've grasped the key points.

- **Acknowledge emotions:** Repeat and acknowledge the other person's emotions to show that you're paying attention to their feelings.

By incorporating these strategies thoughtfully, you can improve your communication skills and build stronger, more meaningful connections with others.

The Importance of Flexibility

Relationships are dynamic. Your ADHD mind is dynamic. So, why do we assume our strategies don't have to be? It's vital to embrace flexibility when it comes to your relationship tools and techniques. What does that mean? It means that you shouldn't expect a one-size-fits-all approach. There is no one right answer. Instead, you should be willing to switch approaches when something isn't working. As the relationship changes over time, you might need new tools and strategies to match the evolved relationship. When you remain flexible and keep trying, improvement will continue to occur, even when you might not notice it.

A couple of years ago, I worked with a client, Hannah, who had just started dating a guy she used to be friends with for years. The relationship transitioned into something more on its own, and they were both quite surprised when they learned that they liked each other as more than just friends. However, Hannah struggled to make the switch in her mind. While they were romantic, she still treated him as she did her other male friends. She listened to his stories the same way she always had: while on her phone. When he expressed to her that it upset him, she was taken aback.

"I haven't changed," she told me, quite defensively. "But your relationship did," I responded.

As relationships grow and change, you will need to adjust and incorporate new tools to ensure that the relationship continues to grow and remain healthy. Don't try to hold on to tools that no longer work. Instead, be open to change and be flexible with the tools you choose to put in your toolbox. Something that can help with that is the personalized progress tracker.

Personalized Progress Tracker

All the tools and techniques we've discussed over the last five chapters have one thing in common: they work even better once they're customized. It's the same with these relationship tools. The better you customize it and make it your own, the better it will work for you. You can personalize your techniques and tools by getting to know your social and relationship dynamics a bit better. For example, ask yourself a couple of questions so you'll understand what your relationship goals are and why previous tools haven't been as successful as you'd hoped. Here are a few questions to ask yourself:

- What types of social situations make you feel most comfortable or connected?

- What behaviors or habits have caused friction in your past relationships?

- What are your biggest communication challenges?

- What are your expectations of communication in relationships?

- What type of social situations make you feel anxious or overwhelmed?

- What communication behaviors have caused fractions in your past relationships?

To help you keep track of which tools and techniques you've tried (and which ones were more successful than the others), you can make use of the personalized progress tracker. What is that? It's a simple table that allows you to see your goals, the tools you've tried, and how well they did or didn't work. The goal of this tracker is not to keep going until you find one perfect strategy but rather to help you become aware that sometimes tools work and sometimes they don't. The key lies in trying new tools and identifying which tools are more likely to work in which situation. Here's an example of such a personalized progress tracker.

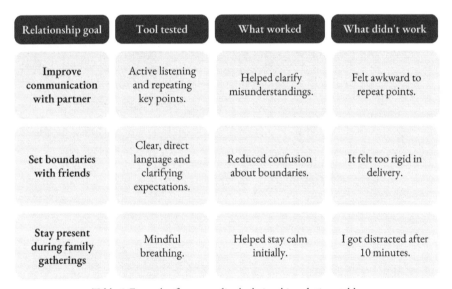

Relationship goal	Tool tested	What worked	What didn't work
Improve communication with partner	Active listening and repeating key points.	Helped clarify misunderstandings.	Felt awkward to repeat points.
Set boundaries with friends	Clear, direct language and clarifying expectations.	Reduced confusion about boundaries.	It felt too rigid in delivery.
Stay present during family gatherings	Mindful breathing.	Helped stay calm initially.	I got distracted after 10 minutes.

Table 6: Example of a personalized relationship solutions table.

Now that you've seen an example in action, it's time to create your own.

Preparing for Relationship Setbacks

Relationships are complex, and setbacks are inevitable. Whether it's an argument with a partner or an awkward interaction at work, it can feel like the end of the world. However, setbacks are normal. While they might not be fun, it's how you recover and stay committed to improvement that really matters. Here's how you can manage and prepare yourself for relationships and social setbacks.

Repair Routine

The first way to prepare yourself for relationship setbacks is by creating a repair routine. What does that mean? It means you have steps in place to ensure that conflict doesn't spiral out of control or that you don't accidentally make the situation worse. If a conversation spirals out of control, it doesn't mean the relationship is doomed. Instead, take a step back, acknowledge the feelings involved, and try again when everyone is in a better headspace. Repairing doesn't have to be perfect; it just needs to be genuine. There are three steps that every repair routine needs to include: Acknowledging emotions, apologizing, and revisiting conversations.

- **Acknowledge emotions:** The first crucial step in creating a repair routine for relationship setbacks is acknowledging your own emotions. As an ADHDer, you might experience a range of emotions after a conflict, such as frustration, anger, sadness, or shame. These emotions can cloud your judgment and hinder effective communication. Therefore, it's essential to take time to identify and acknowledge these emotions within yourself. This can involve journaling, mindfulness exercises, or simply taking a few deep breaths to calm down.

- **Apologize:** Once you've acknowledged your emotions, the next step is to apologize sincerely. This doesn't necessarily mean you were entirely wrong, but it demonstrates a willingness to take responsibility for your role in the conflict. A sincere apology involves acknowledging the impact of your actions on the other person, expressing remorse for any hurt caused, and taking responsibility for your part in the situation. It's crucial to avoid making excuses or blaming the other person. Instead, focus on understanding their perspective and expressing genuine regret for any harm caused.

- **Revisit the conversation:** The final step in this repair routine is to revisit the conversation at a later time when both parties are calm and receptive. When you revisit the conversation, focus on active listening, empathy, and finding common ground to ensure a productive and constructive discussion. Avoid repeating past arguments or getting defensive. Instead, aim to understand the other person's perspective, validate their feelings, and work together to find a solution that works for both of you. This step is crucial for rebuilding trust and strengthening the relationship.

Communication Gaps Are Normal

One of the best ways to prepare yourself for relationship setbacks is to be realistic about them. The truth is that communication gaps are normal. Even neurotypicals experience communication gaps, and that's totally okay. It's part of being human beings and having individual minds and thought processes. However, with ADHD, these gaps tend to be even wider due to distractibility and impulsivity. That's also totally okay. It's nothing to be ashamed of, but it's crucial to be aware of. It's normal to experience these communication gaps, which is why you should have strategies in place to address them when they occur.

A client of mine, Lisa, struggled with listening to other people's stories without getting distracted. Her husband loves playing computer games with immersive storylines, and he enjoys telling her about the games he's been playing. She loves listening to him, especially since she knows it's something he's passionate about. However, she finds it really challenging to keep track of the stories. One moment, she's still listening, and the next, it's wandering off. Her husband picks up on her distractions and then asks, "Are you still with me?" to which she nods and pretends. This makes him feel like she's not actually interested in his stories.

What was my advice to her? Stop pretending. She didn't need another tool to help her listen to stories. All she needed, and all her husband wanted, was honesty. Now, when she drifts off and misses a sentence or five, she stops her husband and asks him to please repeat what he just said. Honesty builds trust, and the right people will appreciate your effort to stay engaged.

Advocating for Understanding

To build a strong relationship, you need to let the other person into your world. What does that mean? It means allowing your partner into your world of ADHD, helping them to understand what ADHD really is and how it's affecting you. At the beginning of the relationship, you might start with broader explanations and positive traits. For example, you can give ADHD credit for your witty remark that made them laugh. In a more long-term relationship, you can begin to focus on your specific challenges and collaborative problem-solving. For example, you can ask for their help in creating a system to keep track of bills so you don't miss important payments.

Educating others on ADHD needs to be simple. They don't have to be able to write an essay on the topic once they're finished speaking. They simply need to have a better understanding of how it can impact people than they had before. Breaking down the complexities of the conditions into more relatable and empathetic ways will dismantle stereotypes and foster more supportive relationships. If you want to explain ADHD to your partner without sounding like a professor, you can say something like this: "When I forget important details, it's not because I don't care, but because my brain prioritizes information differently. Here's how we can work together to improve this." That way, you help them see how your brain is different, and you invite them to join you in the process.

Advocating is a crucial part of the journey, so don't be scared to invite people into the process. You don't have to use all the right words and scientific explanations; all you need is your personal experience. The more relatable the explanation, the more likely others are to understand and provide you with the support you need. Keep this in mind as we embark on the next chapter, which is all about managing ADHD at work.

Chapter Takeaway

- ADHD can greatly impact relationships, both platonic and romantic.

- The impact of ADHD on relationships is like a ripple in the water that expands into something much larger.

- Being flexible with your tools is vital since it needs to be personal to you.

- There will be setbacks, and that's okay. The important thing is that you keep going.

Chapter 6

Navigating Workplace Dynamics With ADHD

"People with ADHD often have a special feel for life, a way of seeing right into the heart of matters, while others have to reason their way methodically."

Edward M. Hallowell

I never realized how hard it was to navigate the workplace as an AD-HDer until I started working. I thought college was hard, but it was nothing compared to the workplace. I felt like a toddler going to daycare for the first time: tired and confused, and I just wanted my mom. I distinctly remember one morning about three months ago, forcing myself out of bed and thinking, *I don't think I can do this for another 40 years.* It was overwhelming getting used to all the new people, the office space, and the thousands of systems in place. I remember asking my supervisor for permission to record our conversations because it felt impossible to remember anything.

I'm sure I'm not the only one who experienced working for the first time as such a traumatic experience. In fact, I've since helped many ADHDers with this transition. Whether it's your first time entering the workplace or if you've been around the block a few times, ADHD will always impact your workplace dynamic. The important thing is that we're prepared to do something about it and set ourselves up for success. Unfortunately, we live in a world that wasn't created with the ADHD brain in mind. There are countless systems everywhere we go that challenge how we are wired, and it's no different in the workplace.

ADHD manifests differently in the workplace depending on job roles, environments, and individual traits. To implement strategies that work, we need to be aware of this truth and be willing to create our own systems. We can't blame ADHD for poor work performance, and we can't expect someone else to make the adjustments for us. A big part of entering the workplace as an ADHDer means you need to be confident in advocating for yourself.

In this chapter, we'll look at the reality of ADHD in the workplace, the types of jobs, and their impact on someone who has ADHD. We'll then explore a few ADHD strategies for the workplace that actually work and what process to follow to ensure that every ADHDer finds their own work style. We'll also explore how ADHD can influence workplace relationships and leadership. Lastly, we'll take a look at how you can tailor your workplace to your specific needs and how to prepare yourself for possible setbacks. So, are you ready to elevate your workplace and find your groove? Let's jump right in!

The Reality of ADHD in the Workplace

Usually, when I speak to managers and neurotypical employees about the reality of ADHD in the workplace, they are completely shocked. Most people assume that ADHD struggles end when you're a child. At most, they think it only influences your ability to sit still. The reality is that it's much worse than that. I presently spoke to a young woman who had started her own small business. While she loved the freedom and seeing the fruits of her creativity, some days, she found it impossible to sit down and work on her admin. "My brain is fine, but it's like my legs are incapable of allowing me to sit still, to the point where it's painful," she shared with me.

Many people assume that fidgeting or restlessness is a silly habit or something ADHDers do subconsciously. But restlessness can tank your productivity. I often use the treadmill as an example to help neurotypicals understand: Asking someone with ADHD to sit still is like putting you on a treadmill and expecting you not to move with the treadmill, but also, you're not allowed to fall off. It doesn't seem possible, does it? When you're compelled to move, you can't just *ignore it away*. Struggles that ADHDers experience in the workplace include difficulty with focus, meeting deadlines, and navigating workplace relationships. Here's a closer look at a few other ADHD struggles you might commonly experience at work.

- **Zoning out:** Have you ever been in a meeting and afterward you can't remember a single thing that was said? You look at the notes you attempted to take during the meeting, only to find your shopping and the same doodles you've been drawing since you were in high school. ADHD makes it hard to sustain focus on a single task, especially for an extended period of time. Minds can wander easily to thoughts, daydreams, and unrelated tasks. Zoning out can lead to missed deadlines and incomplete work. For example, during a presentation, you might find your mind drifting to a personal problem, a song lyric you're obsessed with, or literally anything other than what the presentation is about.

- **Distractions and the fear of missing out:** ADHDers get easily distracted, and then that distraction is all they can focus on.

Something as simple as a notification, a coworker's conversation nearby, or a sudden noise can completely derail focus. Additionally, the impulsive nature of ADHD can also lead to the constant urge to check emails, social media, and other distractions, scared that you'll miss something important. For example, while working on a report, you hear two coworkers talk about your favorite TV show. All you want is to be part of the conversation and share your thoughts with them, making it impossible to focus on the task at hand.

- **Sensory overload:** ADHDers are highly sensitive to sensory input. Loud noises, bright lights, strong smells, or even uncomfortable textures can be overwhelming and distracting (which is why a kitchen microwave is literally the worst piece of equipment in an office). But sensory overload isn't just an *ick*. It can lead to a complete shutdown, making it impossible to concentrate and triggering anxiety. For example, a fluorescent light flickering in an office can be intensely distracting for ADHDers. One moment, you're still working; the next, you're singing a song that matches the beat of the flickering light.

- **Dopamine-draining tasks:** ADHDers rely on strong dopamine responses for motivation and focus. Repetitive, monotonous tasks that don't provide a sense of novelty or challenge can be extremely draining, as they don't trigger the same dopamine release. This can lead to procrastination, avoidance, and a general lack of engagement. For example, data entry or proofreading, while important, can be incredibly tedious for ADHDers. The lack of immediate reward or stimulation can make it difficult to stay motivated and complete the task.

Unfortunately, this often makes managers and CEOs question whether it's worth it to hire someone with ADHD. It absolutely is! ADHDers possess strength in roles where they are allowed to be creative and solve problems. Even though they might struggle in certain types of jobs, in other roles, ADHDers can thrive. A study found that individuals with ADHD were more likely to be employed in creative fields such as art, design, and writing (Mutti-Driscoll, 2025). These fields often value innovative thinking and the ability to generate new ideas, which can be strengths for individuals with ADHD. However, the same study found that individuals with ADHD were less likely to be employed in fields that require high levels of attention to detail and routine tasks, such as accounting or data entry. With this in mind, let's take a look at the different types of jobs and their impact on someone with ADHD.

Types of Jobs and Their Impact

Finding the right job with ADHD can be a significant challenge due to the core symptoms of ADHD. It can be hard to stay organized and motivated during the application process, which can involve meticulous resume writing, researching companies, and preparing for interviews. Not to mention the interview itself and impressing complete strangers. However, it's not impossible to find a job that you enjoy, but in order to do so, you need to be aware of which jobs are more likely to suit an ADHD mind and which ones might be more challenging.

Repetitive Jobs

A repetitive job involves performing the same tasks over and over and over and over and over again. These tasks are often simple and don't require a lot of variation or decision-making. They're also boring, come to think of it, which is why the ADHD brain would rather do anything else than a repetitive job. Examples of repetitive jobs include factory workers, data entry clerks, and warehouse workers. The biggest struggle for ADHDers in repetitive roles is maintaining focus on the monotonous tasks.

There are a few small things you can implement to make repetitive jobs more fun and ADHD-friendly. One of the most successful tools for making receptive jobs survivable is to gamify them. Gamification is the process of applying game-like elements to non-game contexts to increase engagement, motivation, and productivity.

An ADHD friend of mine loves the television game show *Survivor*. As a mom of four who also takes care of her parents, her day consists of repetitive tasks. From hanging the laundry to making dinner for eight people, everything seems repetitive. So, she started creating her own *Survivor* challenges at home. Throughout the day, she has to compete for ingredients that she uses to make dinner. If she can hang that load of laundry in ten minutes, she gets to choose a protein of her choice. Turning it into a game has helped her to remain engaged and positive.

You can gamify your repetitive job by

- creating a points and reward system.

- using a leaderboard to track your (and perhaps your colleagues') progress.

- implementing levels and achievements.

- using storytelling and narrative.

- implementing progress bars and visualizations.

- applying friendly competition.

Creative Roles

A creative role involves using imagination, innovation, and artistic expression to generate new ideas, concepts, or solutions. These roles often require individuals to think outside the box, experiment with different approaches, and craft something new. Creative roles are ideal for a majority of ADHDers as they leverage hyperfocus and out-of-the-box thinking. However, it's not all sunshine and rainbows. Balancing creativity with deadlines can be very tricky for ADHDers. You can't rush art, right? Well, turns out you kind of have to when it's your livelihood. Hyperfocus can often cause ADHDers to zoom in on perfecting one aspect of a task while the rest has to wait and then fall behind schedule. For example, an ADHD graphic designer might spend hours obsessing over finding the perfect font while neglecting the more important tasks.

To manage creativity and deadlines, you have to implement strategies such as setting timers, using reminders, and collaborating with peers to keep you on track and efficient.

Leadership and Decision-Making Roles

ADHDers excel at quick decision-making and adaptability due to their ability to process information rapidly and draw quick connections. Therefore, they can make excellent leaders, especially in a crisis that requires creativity and innovation. However, there are also many challenges that ADHDers experience in leadership roles. Managing impulsivity and enduring follow-through can be a difficult task. In a crisis, quick thinking is crucial, but leadership also requires well-thought-out decisions that consider the long-term effect.

To manage the balance in leadership, ADHDers can rely on tools to support them with decision-making and implement a management team that can provide counsel. ADHDers can also use project management software to track progress and set up regular check-ins with the rest of the team.

Take Emily as an example. Emily is a CEO with ADHD, known for her visionary leadership and ability to inspire her employees. Her creative thinking and out-of-the-box ideas drive innovation within the company. While she may struggle with traditional management styles, she fosters a collaborative environment where her team feels empowered to contribute their own unique perspectives. She delegates routine administrative tasks and focuses on building strong relationships with her team, creating a culture of trust and open communication.

It might not be easy to find your workstyle at first but don't give up. If it's a job or a role you really want, work together with others to find systems that work for you. You can also rely on some of the following ADHD strategies to help you manage your ADHD symptoms at work.

Finding Your Work Style

Since there are so many things that can impact your work as an ADHDer, finding a work style that works for you can be a difficult monster to slay. That doesn't mean you shouldn't try, though. There are many things to consider when it comes to work style and which strategies are effective, which means you'll need to keep track of the strategies you've tried and whether they were helpful or not. To help you on this journey of finding your work style, ask yourself some questions to reflect on and find insight into what tends to work for you or not. Here are a few questions to get you started:

- What tasks do you find easiest to focus on, and why?

- In what kind of work environment (quiet, dynamic, collaborative) do you feel most productive?

- What types of tasks drain your energy, and how can you manage or delegate them?

- What part of the day do you feel the most productive?

- What distracts you the most when you work?

- How do you prefer to receive and process information?

- What type of rewards or incentives motivate you?

- How well do you handle pressure and stress?

To keep track of your findings, you can use a personalized work tools tracker. This is a very simple table that will allow you to see the challenges you're experiencing at work, as well as the tools you've tried, what worked and didn't work, and future alternatives. Here's an example of what it might look like.

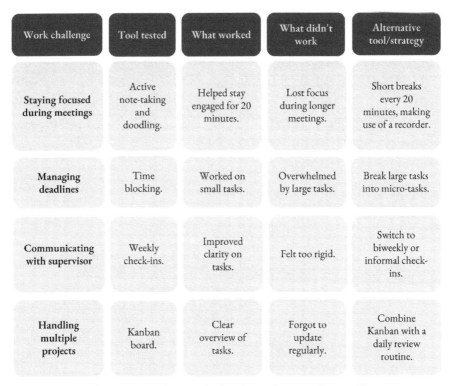

Work challenge	Tool tested	What worked	What didn't work	Alternative tool/strategy
Staying focused during meetings	Active note-taking and doodling.	Helped stay engaged for 20 minutes.	Lost focus during longer meetings.	Short breaks every 20 minutes, making use of a recorder.
Managing deadlines	Time blocking.	Worked on small tasks.	Overwhelmed by large tasks.	Break large tasks into micro-tasks.
Communicating with supervisor	Weekly check-ins.	Improved clarity on tasks.	Felt too rigid.	Switch to biweekly or informal check-ins.
Handling multiple projects	Kanban board.	Clear overview of tasks.	Forgot to update regularly.	Combine Kanban with a daily review routine.

Table 7: Example of a personalized workspace dynamics solutions table.

Now that you know how to use the personalized work tools tracker, it is time for you to create your own.

Workplace Relationships

Workplace relationships can be tricky for everyone, not just ADHDers. Sometimes, personalities clash, conflict arises, or you don't agree with someone else's work ethic. It's okay not to be best friends with everyone at your work, but you should at least try to keep relationships healthy. For a workplace relationship to be considered healthy, it must consist of mutual respect, open communication, and a shared commitment to achieving common goals. It involves treating colleagues with kindness and consideration and actively listening to their perspectives.

However, ADHDers might find this a little tricky. Impulsivity can lead to unintentional outbursts of off-the-cuff remarks that can offend colleagues. Furthermore, inattentiveness can result in missed social cues, forgotten commitments, or a perceived lack of engagement, which can strain relationships with coworkers and supervisors. While ADHD might come with additional struggles with regard to workplace relationships, it's vital to focus and become aware of the struggles so you can find an appropriate solution.

Boss-Employee Dynamics

As you might be aware, ADHDers tend to struggle with time management and prioritization. This can lead to a pattern of starting tasks at the last minute, which might be perceived as procrastination by their boss. Even though the behavior isn't always intentional, it can create a difficult dynamic between the ADHDer and the employer. Similarly, disorganization might be seen as laziness or a lack of effort. Due to messy desks, missed deadlines, or difficulty keeping track of tasks, bosses might mistakenly interpret the ADHDers' behavior as a careless attitude. Due to the stigmas surrounding ADHD, many ADHDers prefer to disclose their condition to their employers, which can create a significant barrier to open communication and understanding. Without this open dialogue, bosses may continue to misinterpret ADHD behaviors as laziness or incompetence, leading to increased stress and reduced self-esteem for the employee.

On the other side of the coin, the ADHD employee might live in a constant state of fear of being judged or misunderstood, which can lead to significant stress and anxiety for ADHDers in the workplace. This can negatively impact their overall well-being and decrease productivity, adding even more stress and pressure to the mix. Repeating negative feedback or perception of laziness can erode an individual's self-esteem and confidence.

This can make it even harder to overcome the challenges of ADHD in their role.

This reminds me of a young woman I worked with a few years ago, Cara. Cara thrived on creativity and in bursts of intense focus. However, her boss, Mr. Henderson, a stickler for routine and deadlines, constantly criticized her *lack of discipline*. Cara would often miss deadlines, not because she didn't care but because she'd get sidetracked by a new idea, lose track of time, or simply forget to check her email. Mr. Henderson saw this as laziness. He'd leave snide comments on her work, like "Seems like you need to learn to prioritize." Cara felt misunderstood and unfairly judged. The constant criticism eroded her confidence, leading to increased anxiety and a decline in her performance.

One day, Cara reached her breaking point. During a particularly harsh review, she felt a surge of frustration and finally blurted out, "I have ADHD." Mr. Henderson was initially taken aback, but Cara explained that she'd recently been evaluated and was seeking professional help. To her surprise, Mr. Henderson was surprisingly understanding. He admitted he'd been unaware of the challenges of ADHD and expressed a desire to learn more. They started an open dialogue. Cara explained how her mind worked, the challenges she faced, and the strategies that helped her stay focused, such as breaking down tasks, using timers, and minimizing distractions. Mr. Henderson, in turn, adjusted his expectations. He started providing more specific deadlines and encouraged her to check in regularly. He also implemented a system of *checkpoints* to ensure progress on larger projects.

This experience taught both Cara and Mr. Henderson the importance of open communication and understanding. It highlighted that successful workplace relationships are built on trust, empathy, and a willingness to adapt. Even if you don't feel like you have a good relationship with your boss, trust that it is possible and work toward cultivating and maintaining a healthy work relationship with your boss.

Peer-to-Peer Collaboration

Just as ADHD can impact your relationship with your boss, it can also affect your relationship with your peers. ADHDers often struggle with working memory and executive function, making it difficult to remember details like deadlines, meeting times, and assigned tasks. This can create a feeling of unreliability among coworkers. Similarly, ADHDers might find it hard to filter irrelevant information and focus on the most important task for the group. This can lead to misinterpreting priorities and focusing on tasks that might appear selfish from the group's perspective.

Group settings can also be sensory overloading for ADHDers. The constant flow of information, multiple conversations, and distractions can make it difficult to concentrate and participate effectively in group discussions and decision-making processes. This constant overloading might lead to unclear communication, adding to the pressure on peer-to-peer collaboration. To aid in peer-to-peer collaboration, here are a few things to keep in mind:

- **Be upfront about your challenges:** If you're struggling to remember something or need clarification, don't hesitate to ask. It's better to ask for help than to let a misunderstanding fester. Let your colleagues know about your ADHD and how it might affect your work style. This can help manage expectations and build understanding.

- **Break down large tasks:** Divide large projects into smaller, more manageable chunks. This can make the tasks feel less overwhelming and improve your focus. Use reminders on your phone or computer to help you stay on track and avoid missing deadlines or meetings.

- **Make an effort to connect:** Small things like taking time to get to know your colleagues can go a long way. Making an effort is a great way to build rapport and strengthen relationships. Join in on office social events or organize casual get-togethers to build camaraderie.

- **Offer to help:** Be willing to lend a hand to colleagues when needed. This can help build goodwill and show that you're a team player.

- **Communicate your needs:** If you need specific accommodations or support, don't be afraid to ask your manager or HR department. A mentor can also provide guidance, support, and a sounding board for challenges you may face.

- **Use collaboration tools:** Tools such as a Kanban board can be very helpful when you're working together on tasks with your peers. A kanban board will visually track where in the process you are, ensuring that you and your peers are aligned and can constantly check in with one another.

ADHD in Leadership

Since the ADHD mind operates in a non-linear fashion, allowing us to think outside the box, we make great leaders. People often assume leaders should be the best organized and most professional-looking individuals, but that's not always the case. Someone who pushes others to be creative and find new ways to look at things is often exactly what a team needs to thrive. Our creativity can be contagious, allowing us to inspire our team to embrace new ideas and approaches. ADHDers also possess a high level of energy and enthusiasm, which is motivating for team members. Our passion for projects can be infectious, driving our team to achieve ambitious goals. We can also pivot quickly and adjust plans on the fly, ensuring the team stays agile.

However, it's not all good news. ADHD can also cause a few challenges when it comes to leadership roles. One significant hurdle lies in the realm of impulsivity and its impact on decision-making. ADHD can lead to a tendency toward quick, spontaneous decisions without taking the necessary time to think things through and consider the long-term implications. This can manifest in impulsive commitments, shifting priorities, and overlooking potential risks and consequences. Another major hurdle is staying organized and managing multiple projects at the same time. This can be quite overwhelming at times, especially when everyone is looking to you for answers. Difficulties with executive functions can make it hard to prioritize tasks, delegate effectively, and maintain a clear overview of ongoing projects, which can add to the anxiety and overwhelmed feelings.

Leadership comes with challenges for everyone, and it's not a reason for ADHDers not to embrace their role as leaders. Instead, you can look for strategies to help you manage these challenges while also emphasizing your strengths. Here are a few strategies you can rely on:

- **Decision-making frameworks:** There are frameworks you can use that will provide a structured approach to evaluating your options. Examples of these frameworks include SWOT analysis (Strengths, Weaknesses, Opportunities, Threats), cost-benefit analysis, or the Eisenhower Matrix (urgent/important). By forcing a more deliberate consideration of factors and potential outcomes, these frameworks can help mitigate impulsive decisions and ensure that choices are aligned with long-term goals.

- **Project management software:** Tools like Asana, Trello, Mond ay.com, or even simple spreadsheets can be invaluable for ADHD leaders. These tools allow centralized task management, visual progress tracking, and improved delegation.

- **Detail-oriented team members:** You should partner with a detail-oriented team member who can act as a *grounding* influence, ensuring follow-through on ideas and projects. This *check-and-balance* system can be incredibly valuable.

- **Self-reflection periods**: Regular self-reflection (e.g., daily or weekly check-ins) will allow you to assess your progress, identify roadblocks, adjust priorities, and prevent burnout.

You can leverage your strengths while mitigating the challenges associated with ADHD by implementing these strategies. These strategies can improve your decision-making, enhance your organizational skills, and lead to greater success in your leadership roles.

Tailoring Your Work Environment

Since ADHD brains thrive on novelty and variety, it's important that workplace strategies should evolve. Your work style doesn't have to look like anyone else's; it just has to work for you. If a strategy stops working, it's not a failure. It's a sign that you've outgrown it, and it's time to try something new. You have full permission to adapt strategies based on your current job role, work environment, and energy levels. Every day doesn't have to look exactly the same. Instead, make it your own. Reflect each morning on where you're at and what you need to make a success of the day. This reminds me of Chris's story.

For years, Chris struggled as an ADHD leader. His desk was a chaotic mess, deadlines loomed, and his team often felt like he was constantly shifting gears. He tried every productivity app and organization system and even color-coded his calendar. But nothing worked. He felt like a hamster on a wheel, chasing order but never quite getting it. Then, Chris started a new morning ritual. Each morning, before diving into his inbox, he would spend 5–10 minutes reflecting on his day. He asked himself three questions:

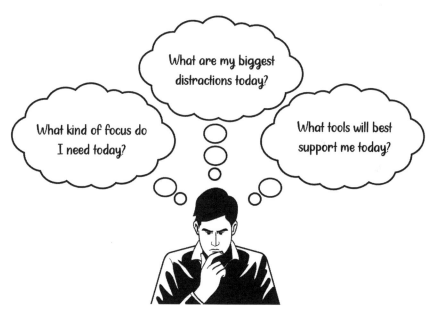

- *What kind of focus do I need today?* Was it deep work for a complex project or quick bursts of attention for a series of meetings?

- *What are my biggest distractions today?* Was it the constant pinging of Slack, the allure of social media, or the tempting siren song of a messy desk?

- *What tools will best support me today?* Do I need the structure of a strict to-do list, the visual clarity of a Kanban board, or the quiet solitude of noise-canceling headphones?

This simple reflection became a game-changer. He realized that his *perfect* productivity system wasn't a one-size-fits-all solution. Some days, he craved the structure of a rigid schedule. On other days, he needed the flexibility to follow his intuition and explore new ideas. This approach not only improved his productivity but also reduced his stress. Instead of feeling constantly overwhelmed by the *shoulds* of productivity, he learned to listen to his brain and choose the tools that best supported his unique needs on any given day.

We can learn from Chris and approach our days the same way. You should tailor your work environment each day to your specific needs. Remember to use your personalized work strategy tracker to help guide you in this process.

Preparing for Workplace Setbacks

Workplace setbacks—missed deadlines, forgotten tasks, or communication breakdowns—are common for individuals with ADHD. It doesn't mean you're a bad employee. It simply means that you're human. The best way to deal with workplace setbacks is to be prepared for when they happen. Here are three things you can do in preparation for setbacks.

Preparing for Workspace Setbacks

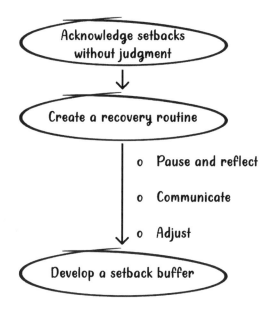

Acknowledge Setbacks Without Judgment

Workplace setbacks are normal. Remember, your ADHD isn't confined to one area of your life. The same struggles you experience at home, you will also experience at work. It's normal to experience these setbacks, and it is crucial to acknowledge them without judgment. Your workplace setbacks don't define your competence as an employee or even as a leader. Missing a deadline or forgetting an important detail doesn't mean you're bad at your job; it means your system needs adjusting. Learn from it, tweak your approach, and keep going.

Create a Recovery Routine

Once you experience the setback, you might be tempted to jump into action or do something to avoid the setback. However, the best way to deal with it is by creating a simple, three-step recovery routine. Here's how:

- **Step 1—Pause and reflect:** Start by acknowledging the setback and the emotions it's triggering. This might include frustration, disappointment, or even anger. It's okay to feel these emotions. Don't try to suppress them. Instead, allow yourself to feel them fully, but don't dwell on them excessively. Reflect on what led to the setback. Instead of focusing solely on the negative, shift your attention to what you can learn from the experience. Viewing setbacks as opportunities for growth can help you develop resilience and move forward more confidently.

- **Step 2—Communicate:** Share your feelings and experiences with a trusted friend, family member, mentor, or therapist. Talking about your challenges can help you gain perspective and receive support. If the setback involved a conflict with a colleague or a misunderstanding with your boss, consider having an open and honest conversation. Explain your perspective calmly and assertively, focusing on finding a resolution and improving future interactions.

- **Step 3—Adjust:** Based on your reflections, create a concrete action plan to address the root causes of the setback. This might involve setting new goals, implementing new strategies, or seeking additional support. Avoid making drastic changes all at once. Start with small, manageable steps and gradually incorporate new habits and routines.

Develop a Setback Buffer

As an ADHDer, you should build in buffers for deadlines and tasks whenever possible. What does that mean? If you tend to underestimate how long tasks take, try setting internal deadlines 24 hours before the actual due date. This will create a buffer, offering some breathing room for unexpected delays. However, it's important to view the internal deadline as the *real* deadline; otherwise, it won't work.

Remember, setbacks are a normal part of life and career development. By preparing for setbacks in these ways, you'll be ready for when they occur. You don't have to be perfect. Just keep learning and growing, and you'll always be a good addition to every team.

Chapter Takeaway

- Different types of jobs can have a different impact on your ADHD mind. Some jobs are more likely to suit someone with ADHD, but that doesn't mean you should limit yourself to only certain roles.

- To find your work style, you need to embrace a trial-and-error approach, constantly updating which tools and strategies work for you.

- Workplace dynamics and relationships can be tough to manage, but not impossible. By being intentional and communicating openly about your struggles, you are more likely to succeed than when you're suffering in silence.

- Setbacks are inevitable, but you can prepare yourself for setbacks to ensure you remain a positive addition to the team.

Chapter 7

Building a Life That Works for You

"Success is not final; failure is not fatal: it is the courage to continue that counts."

Winston Churchill

I can't believe we're already at the last chapter. As you look back on this journey, I want you to imagine each chapter as a set of tools. Chapter one might be screwdrivers, and Chapter three might be spanners. They are all placed before you, ready for you to choose them. But you don't have to choose them all. In fact, you have limited space in your current toolbox. While you can always switch out tools for other ones later, it's time to pick a few to add to your toolbox. Instead of feeling pressure to remember every single tool and technique discussed in this book, make it simpler for yourself and reduce the feeling of overwhelm by choosing a few techniques to focus on first. They are the ones you'll be adding to your toolbox right now.

This toolbox is something you can carry with you to every area of your life, whether it's work or social events. It is always available to you, but it's up to you to take it out and teach yourself how to use it. It might take a few times before you get used to the tools but don't give up. They will allow you to build a life that works for you.

Redefining Success

What does success mean to you? What does it look like? Would you con-sider yourself successful once you've mastered ADHD? Perhaps you'll be successful when ADHD doesn't impact your life anymore. Does success equate to perfection and being flawless? Does it mean you never forget anything, never run later, and never daydream during meetings? Well, I've got some bad news: if that's your measure of success, you'll never succeed. Trust me; I've been there, and it only leads to frustration and even more feelings of failure.

As ADHDers, we tend to be hard on ourselves. We hold ourselves to very high standards because we assume that's what we have to achieve in order to be good enough and make up for all our flaws. But guess what? No one is perfect, and everyone has flaws. We all struggle with things in life, whether we have ADHD or not. Chasing perfection is an endless pursuit. It's like running in quicksand or holding water in your hands.

For many years, I thought success meant never experiencing a setback. So, whenever I inevitably experienced setbacks, I considered myself the oppo-site of successful. I constantly thought I had to start from scratch when things didn't work for me anymore instead of adjusting things slightly. One day, after experiencing a setback, I cried to my husband and told him how I was such a failure. At that moment, my daughter was learning to walk, and he pointed to her and asked, "Do you think she's a failure when she falls on her bum?" I shook my head. "Of course not. She's still learning and growing." In my answer to him, I gave myself an "Aha" moment. Success shouldn't be measured to perfection. We're all still learning and growing, and every step we take, whether forward or backward, is one step closer to reaching our goals.

Traditional definitions of success are often centered on external achievements like a promotion, another degree, or wealth. But all of these can feel quite out of reach or irrelevant for ADHD individuals. So, let's redefine success, shall we? Instead of trying to be perfect at all times, let's focus on what success could mean instead:

- Success is never giving up.

- Success is navigating between the different tools in our arsenal, knowing when to use which.

- Success means knowing when you need a break and when you need to push on.

- Success is being kind to yourself and allowing yourself days to reset.

- Success is celebrating the process and finding joy in improvement.

- Success is growing from setbacks and choosing to try again.

- Success is adapting and being flexible.

- Success is building a schedule that works for me today.

Take a moment to redefine what success means to you. What needs to happen for you to consider this meeting a success? How can you embrace a mindset of success that isn't linked to perfection? What makes you feel accomplished and proud? What small win has recently brought you joy? Remember, you are strong and capable, even when you experience setbacks.

Integrating ADHD Strategies Into Everyday Life

In front of you, you have tons of tools to choose from. The best toolbox consists of a variety of tools. To build a life that works for you, you need to find a way to combine emotional regulation techniques, productivity and organization systems, and relationship tools into one harmonizing toolbox. Integrating these strategies means using them together to combat the interconnected challenges of ADHD. For example, emotional regulation techniques like mindfulness can reduce the stress that hinders productivity, while relationship tools such as active listening foster support systems that reinforce other strategies. It's all about finding the combinations that work for you.

Jamie, an ADHD adult, struggled to maintain focus at work, and he also neglected self-care. After following the steps in this book, he created his toolbox and implemented a combination of strategies. Now, every morning, he begins with a grounding exercise, followed by using a visual board to organize his priorities and set boundaries for his personal time. In doing this, he's found a way to achieve a sustainable balance. His transformation showcases the importance of approaching ADHD holistically, including tools to effectively manage your ADHD in all areas of your life.

Celebrating Progress

Celebrating progress is a powerful way to reinforce positive behavior and your new view of success. When you celebrate how far you've come, instead of focusing on how far you still need to go, you will feel motivated instead of overwhelmed. Acknowledging even the smallest victories, like completing a task on time or staying focused for 10 minutes, can create a sense of accomplishment that fuels further progress. We've already spoken about celebrating the progress in other sections on this journey, so let's put it into practice right now.

What are three things you can cele-brate right in this moment? Perhaps you can celebrate reading this book so far already? Maybe you've completed a task you've been dreading for weeks this morning? Or maybe you simply went to bed at a decent time for once! All of these are wonderful reasons to celebrate your progress on this ADHD journey of yours. You can even create a celebration 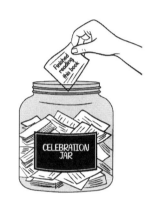 jar celebrating your progress. What is a celebration jar? It's a jar you keep, and every time you have something to celebrate, you write it down on a piece of paper and add it to the jar. Over time, this jar will become a tangible representative of your achievements, offering a motivation boost during challenging moments. Speaking of challenging times, let's take a look at how to navigate the ups and downs of ADHD life.

Navigating Life's Ups and Downs

As you know very well, life with ADHD is inherently unpredictable, and setbacks are inevitable. It's like being strapped to a rollercoaster with no idea of the twists and turns coming up ahead. The changes can come quickly and without warning, leaving you drained and frustrated. There's no map you can use to navigate these ups and downs of life; it's part of what makes us human. But that doesn't mean you should just surrender and allow yourself to be thrown around by the ups and downs. Instead, if you learn to navigate it, you'll find your rhythm in the ups and the downs. In other words, you'll recover faster, learn more, and be resilient. Here are three things to keep in mind while trying to navigate the ups and downs of life.

Embrace Imperfection

Sasha, a vibrant whirlwind of ideas and energy, always felt like her ADHD was a superpower waiting to be unleashed. She dreamed of a perfectly organized life—a meticulously planned schedule, a pristine workspace, and a mind that effortlessly focused on one task at a time. She devoured self-help books on ADHD management, eager to unlock the *secret* to a perfectly balanced life. She bought sleek planners, invested in noise-canceling headphones, and even tried neurofeedback. For a while, it felt like magic. Her to-do list shrank, her desk gleamed, and she experienced moments of blissful productivity. But the perfection she craved remained elusive. Distractions inevitably crept in.

One day, while lamenting over a spilled coffee stain on her pristine desk, a thought struck her. Was this constant striving for perfection actually hindering her joy? Was she so focused on achieving an *ideal* life that she was missing the beauty of the present moment? Sasha began to embrace the chaos. She learned to accept that her mind would wander, that distractions were inevitable, and that sometimes, the most creative ideas emerged from the unexpected. She started to view her ADHD not as a deficit but as a unique perspective, a source of boundless energy and creativity.

She discovered that ADHD management wasn't about achieving a flawless, robotic existence. It was about finding strategies that helped her navigate her unique brain, work with her strengths, and cultivate self-compassion. It was about accepting the messy, vibrant reality of her life and finding joy in the unexpected twists and turns along the way. Just like Sasha, some days you'll feel like you're nailing it; other days, not so much. That's okay. Progress isn't about getting it right every time. It's about showing up, trying again, and learning along the way.

Develop a Reset Plan for Bad Days

Bad days will come, and there's nothing you can do to prevent them. But that doesn't mean you should let it ruin your week. A bad hour doesn't have to change into a bad day, and a bad day doesn't have to turn into a bad week. Here's how you can develop a simple reset plan for bad days:

- **Step 1—Acknowledge the setback without judgment:** After a challenging day, it's crucial to acknowledge the setbacks without self-criticism. This involves recognizing that things didn't go according to plan and accepting these feelings without judgment. Instead of dwelling on what went wrong, focus on understanding the obstacles faced. For example, let's say you planned to complete an important project but ended up procrastinating all day, getting lost in social media, and tackling random, low-priority tasks instead. Instead of beating yourself up with thoughts like *"Why am I like this? I wasted an entire day!"*, take a step back. Ask yourself: *What got in my way?* Did distractions derail your focus? Did fatigue or emotional overwhelm impact your productivity? Maybe you were mentally drained and needed more breaks than you allowed yourself. Recognizing these factors without self-blame is key to moving forward constructively.

- **Step 2—Identify one small action:** Often, after a difficult day, the thought of tackling a to-do list can feel overwhelming. This step focuses on breaking down that overwhelming feeling by identifying just one small, achievable action. It could be something as simple as tidying up your workspace, preparing a quick and easy meal, or even just spending 15 minutes reading a book. The goal is to regain a sense of control and accomplishment, no matter how small. This small victory could provide a much-needed boost of motivation and confidence for the next day.

- **Step 3—Set a new, manageable goal for the day:** Instead of dwelling on the unfinished tasks from the previous day, this step involves re-evaluating your to-do list and setting a new, manageable goal for the following day. This might involve prioritizing the most essential tasks, or even reducing the overall number of tasks on the list. Time blocking can also be helpful in this step, scheduling specific time slots for tasks to maintain focus and minimize distractions.

If you've had a rough week and everything feels out of control, start small. Make a list of three things you can do today, no matter how small they seem. Small steps lead to bigger wins.

Prepare for Periods of Low Motivation

ADHD can cause periods of low motivation that can feel overwhelming and even lead to burnout. Remember that these periods are temporary and that there are strategies to overcome them. These periods of low motivation are not a reflection of our worth or abilities. They are a symptom of ADHD, and it's important to approach them with self-compassion. Instead of beating ourselves up for not being productive, we can acknowledge that we're experiencing a dip in motivation and that it's okay to take a break or adjust our expectations. On low-motivation days, lower the bar.

Instead of aiming for perfection, aim for done. Progress matters more than how it looks.

Finding motivation when we're struggling can feel like an uphill battle. However, here's a reminder of a few techniques discussed in this book that can help you keep going and remain motivated.

- **Break down tasks:** Divide large tasks into smaller, more manageable steps. This can make them feel less daunting and increase our sense of accomplishment.

- **Reward yourself:** Celebrate small victories, no matter how insignificant they might seem. Rewarding yourself with a celebration can help reinforce positive behavior and motivate us to keep going.

- **Find a support system:** Connect with others who understand ADHD. Sharing experiences and challenges can provide valuable support and encouragement.

As this journey together is coming to an end, there's one crucial thing you should always remember: You are building a life that evolves. Your life is a work in progress, and so are your strategies. Keep checking in with yourself, keep adapting, and keep moving forward—one step at a time.

Chapter Takeaway

- Traditional definitions of success can be harmful to ADHDers. That's why we should redefine success as more accessible, more positive things.

- Integrating ADHD strategies into your life means approaching things holistically and combining different tools to create the best strategy for you. Don't be scared to mix and match tools from different areas of your life.

- Celebrating progress is essential, and a celebration jar is a great way to have a tangible reflection of your success.

- Life will throw you ups and downs, but you can navigate it by embracing imperfection, developing a reset plan, and preparing for periods of low motivation.

Note from the Author

Hi there,

Yes, you made it! You've come a long way, and I am proud of you. This was no small feat, so give yourself a pat on the back.

First of all, before you go to the conclusion, don't forget to grab the free material offered at the beginning of this book if you are interested. It might help you on your journey moving forward. Here is the QR code again:

(https://amy-harper.kit.com/fca05047ec)

Second, if you want to know more about my other titles or explore other ADHD content and tools, please visit me at:

- **www.pluralcreations.com/amyharper**

Or send me an email directly:

- **amy.harper@pluralcreations.com**

Last but certainly not least, I highly value your opinion, and I'd like to hear your feedback. I humbly ask that you **consider writing an honest review** about your experience. Your act of kindness will help me immensely, and it will also help other readers. Even a few sentences can make a huge difference, and if you're really feeling up to it, a photo or video review would mean the world. Your support will never be forgotten.

Thank you in advance!

Just scan the QR code below:

Remember, you're capable of amazing things, and I'm here rooting for you every step of the way.

Amy Harper

Conclusion

Moving Forward With Confidence

"If you can't fly then run, if you can't run then walk, if you can't walk then crawl, but whatever you do you have to keep moving forward."

Martin Luther King Jr.

L ook where you are: at the end of this book! You finished reading it, which I know isn't an easy task for an ADHDer. I am incredibly proud of you, and before you go your own way, I have a few more golden nuggets I'd like to encourage you with. Don't worry, I won't go all sappy on you. I promised you I wouldn't sugarcoat things, and I'm not about to start now, so here's something you need to be prepared for: On this journey, you will experience setbacks. You'll be faced with challenges that seem impossible to overcome, and you might even try techniques that don't work for you. But guess what? That's part of life, and by moving forward after setbacks, you'll acquire resilience.

The best gift you can give yourself is to stop viewing setbacks as failures. Missed a deadline? That's okay. Instead of beating yourself up over it, why not view it as an opportunity to revisit the systems you have in place and tweak them to prevent a missed deadline in the future? As an ADHDer, you should normalize a trial-and-error nature to your management strategies. In other words, expect new methods not to be successful the first time. Expect them to shed some light, but still have things that require change before they work for you. That way, you won't be disappointed when the method doesn't work immediately, which means you won't be tempted to give up. Instead, you'll think, *Of course, it wasn't going to work, but now I know why, and I can adapt it accordingly.* Remember, every small step is a forward contribution to long-term growth.

To help you keep moving forward, here are two things for you to rely on.

Stay Connected

One of the most underrated ADHD methods is having someone to support and encourage you. Most things in life are easier when you have someone with you. Whether they're actually able to help or simply be there for moral support, it can do wonders for your progress to have someone that you're connected to. This is especially true if the other person understands ADHD and can relate to your struggles and victories. The goal isn't to compare your struggles to see who has it worse or to use your struggles as excuses, but rather to encourage and support one another.

When I have a bad day, and none of my methods seem to help, an iced coffee with my ADHD best friend always helps me. Does it solve my problems? Not directly. But she also encourages me to keep going. She celebrates how far I've come and reminds me of the progress when it seems invisible. Above all, she's a safe space. She listens without judgment as I share how I forgot to order my husband's birthday present or showed up late to pick up my children from school. Most of the time, sharing my *failures* with her allows me to laugh about them and move forward without judgment.

Do you have someone you can rely on for support? If not, I highly recommend joining an ADHD support group, whether in person or online. This way, you'll have someone to share insights with, you'll find encouragement, and remain motivated to keep going.

Keep Learning

Other than remaining connected, you should also adopt a mindset of lifelong learning. Even as you finish this book, don't see it as the end. This is only the beginning. ADHD is a lifelong journey, and as you change and new methods are developed, you'll learn more about your mind and how to manage it effectively. The most important thing is to remain curious about your ADHD. Don't assume you know it all and have all the answers. There's still so much to uncover and explore. By remaining curious about your unique brain, you'll ensure preparedness for whatever might come your way. You can continue learning by reading blogs, listening to podcasts, and studying other books on the topic. Some books I recommend include

- *Taking Charge of ADHD* by Russell A. Barkley

- *You Mean I'm Not Lazy, Stupid or Crazy?!* by Kate Kelly and Peggy Ramundo

- *Organizing Solutions for People* With ADHD by Susan Pinsky

- *The ADHD Effect on Marriage* by Melissa Orlov

- *The Mindfulness Prescription for Adult ADHD* by Lidia Zylowska

So, What Now?

What happens now? First of all, throw yourself a mini-celebration for finishing this book. Then, take what you've learned and begin to apply it to your life. You have to make it practical. You can have all the knowledge in the world, but without application, it won't lead to change. It's up to you where to begin. You don't have to start with the first methods mentioned in the book. Instead, begin with the method that excites you the most. You can also begin small. Don't try to change your whole life in one day. Begin with one or two techniques and take it from there. As you find the sweet spot with your applied methods, begin to add other techniques as well.

You've got this.

Now go take that first step—whatever it looks like for you.

Acknowledgements

This book wouldn't exist without the unwavering support and patience of my better half. Through countless late nights, endless revisions, and moments of self-doubt, you stood by me—offering encouragement when I needed it most. Your belief in my work kept me going, your feedback sharpened my vision, and your quiet strength carried me through. Thank you for being my critic, my cheerleader, my sounding board, and my steady foundation throughout this journey.

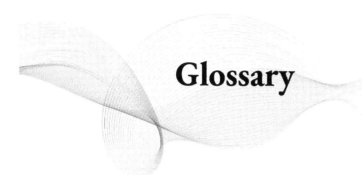

Glossary

ADHDer: This is a friendly way to say someone who has ADHD (Attention-Deficit/Hyperactivity Disorder). It's like using *runner* for someone who runs or *musician* for someone who plays music. ADHDers often prefer this more casual term since it feels less medical or scientific and more *normal*.

Distractability: Have you ever been super focused on something, only to get completely sidetracked by a squirrel (or a shiny object, or a sudden urge to reorganize your sock drawer)? That's distractibility in action! It's our ADHD brains' tendency to get easily pulled away from what we're supposed to be doing.

Dopamine: This neurotransmitter plays a crucial role in motivation, reward, pleasure, and movement. For ADHDers, the dopamine system is dysregulated, leading to challenges with focus, motivation, and experiencing pleasure. This can manifest as difficulty with attention, impulsivity, and finding activities rewarding enough to sustain effort.

Emotional dysregulation: Think of it like a rollercoaster of emotions. With emotional dysregulation, it's hard to control those ups and downs. Feelings can feel intense and overwhelming, and it might be tough to calm yourself down when things get tough.

Emotional regulation: Imagine having a toolbox for your emotions—that's what emotional regulation is all about. It allows you to manage your feelings in a healthy way. This could mean finding ways to calm down when you're feeling stressed, or learning how to express your feelings without getting overwhelmed.

Executive function: A set of mental skills that help us plan, organize, focus, and manage our time and behavior. These skills include attention, working memory, problem-solving, self-control, and flexibility. In ADHDers, executive function skills may be underdeveloped or less efficient, leading to challenges in areas like schoolwork, relationships, and daily life.

Fight-or-flight response: This is our body's natural alarm system. When we feel threatened (even if it's not a real danger), our bodies go into overdrive. Our heart races, we might feel panicky, and we're ready to either fight or run away.

Hyperactive: This term describes excessive physical activity, restlessness, and difficulty sitting still. In the context of ADHD, hyperactivity can manifest as constant fidgeting, squirming, tapping, excessive talking, and difficulty remaining seated during class or other situations that require sustained attention. Not everyone with ADHD experiences hyperactivity.

Hyperfocus: A state of intense concentration and deep immersion in a specific activity, often characterized by narrowed attention, loss of track of time, and reduced awareness of surroundings. It can also be accompanied by increased productivity and enhanced motivation. For example, when you open your cupboard to look for a jersey, and 30 minutes later, you're reorganizing your entire closet, wearing a hat you forgot you had and not the jersey you went there for. But at least your closet is now clean and color-coded.

Hyper-fixation: This is when you get super into something and can't seem to stop thinking about it or doing it. It's like your brain is stuck on repeat! While it can be awesome for getting things done, it can also make it hard to focus on other important stuff.

Inattention: This is one of the core symptoms of ADHD. It refers to the difficulty in sustaining focus and attention on a task or activity. This can manifest as easy distractibility, trouble following instructions, forgetfulness, and difficulty organizing tasks. ADHDers with inattention may appear daydreamy, lose track of time, and have trouble completing assignments.

Intrusive thoughts: Unwanted and unwelcome thoughts that pop into your head unexpectedly. They can be anything from silly to scary, and they can feel really annoying or even distressing.

Impulsivity: This is characterized by difficulty controlling urges and acting without thinking. Impulsivity can manifest in various ways, such as interrupting others, blurting out answers, engaging in risky behaviors, and difficulty waiting for turns.

Neurotransmitters: These are chemical messengers that transmit signals between neurons in the brain. These signals are essential for all brain functions, including attention, movement, mood, and learning.

Neurodivergent: This is a fancy word for having a brain that works differently from the *typical* way. People who are neurodivergent might have conditions like ADHD, autism, dyslexia, or others. It's all about celebrating the unique ways our brains are wired!

Neurotypical: This refers to people whose brains develop and function in a way that's considered *typical* or *average* in society.

Norepinephrine: This is a special chemical in our brains that helps us focus, pay attention, and feel alert. Think of it like the brain's own energy drink!

Procrastination: The art of putting off things you need or want to do, even though you know you should be doing them. It's like your brain is playing a game of "not now!"

Sensory overload: Imagine being at a loud concert with flashing lights and lots of people bumping into you. That's kind of like sensory overload. It happens when our senses (sight, sound, touch, taste, smell) are bombarded with too much information, and it can feel overwhelming and even painful.

Tactile Objects: These are things you can touch and feel! Think squishy stress balls, smooth stones, or even a soft blanket. Tactile objects can help calm us down and bring us back to the present moment when we're feeling overwhelmed.

Time blindness: If you have ADHD, you often lose things, including track of time. Time blindness means you have no idea how long something might take or how long you've already been busy with a task. Five minutes can feel like five hours, and vice versa.

Triggers: These are like hidden landmines for our emotions. They're specific things (like certain sounds, smells, or situations) that can suddenly make us feel anxious, angry, or upset. Once we know our triggers, we can learn to avoid them or develop strategies to cope with them.

References

ADHD, executive functioning, and shame. (2023, February 25). Relational Psych. https://www.relationalpsych.group/articles/adhd-executive-functioning-and-shame

ADHD planners & tools for organization & productivity. (2023, November 22). ADDA - Attention Deficit Disorder Association. https://add.org/adhd-planner/

ADHD quotes: 15 inspirational famous quotations. (2022, April 15). ADDitude. https://www.additudemag.com/slideshows/adhd-famous-quotes-for-a-bad-day/

Boyatzis, R. E., Rochford, K., & Jack, A. I. (2014). Antagonistic neural networks underlying differentiated leadership roles. *Frontiers in Human Neuroscience, 8.* https://doi.org/10.3389/fnhum.2014.00114

Brandman, T., Malach, R., & Simony, E. (2021). The surprising role of the default mode network in naturalistic perception. *Communications Biology, 4*(1). https://doi.org/10.1038/s42003-020-01602-z

Default mode network vs task positive network: ADHD insights. (2024, April 18). Focus Bear. https://www.focusbear.io/blog-post/default-mode-network-vs-task-positive-network-adhd-insights

Dixon, N. (2022, April 13). *Working Memory*. Foothills Academy Society. https://www.foothillsacademy.org/community/articles/working-memory-why-its-important

Dodson, W. (2022, August 24). *ADHD and the epidemic of shame*. ADDitude. https://www.additudemag.com/slideshows/adhd-and-shame/

Hamilton, J. P., Furman, D. J., Chang, C., Thomason, M. E., Dennis, E., & Gotlib, I. H. (2011). Default-mode and task-positive network activity in major depressive disorder: Implications for adaptive and maladaptive rumination. *Biological Psychiatry, 70*(4), 327–333. https://doi.org/10.1016/j.biopsych.2011.02.003

Harris, G. (2020, July 13). *10 fun facts about breathing & the respiratory system*. Gaia. https://www.gaia.com/article/10-interesting-facts-about-breathing?utm_source=Google+Search+Paid&utm_medium=TROAS&utm_campaign=0-dynamic-general-english-EMEA&utm_term=not-applicable&gad_source=1&gclid=Cj0KCQiA4fi7BhC5ARIsAEV1YibdGT1wpvw1lFaUcEvXIs_l18sdudF4MOogoNw9iYLDT9IhRfsPe8QaAnXWEALw_wcB

HCPC. (2021, April 8). *What is reflection?* Health and Care Professions Council. https://www.hcpc-uk.org/standards/meeting-our-standards/reflective-practice/what-is-reflection/

Josel, L. (2024, June 26). *Q: "What mind mapping and study apps for students with ADHD work best?"* ADDitude. https://www.additudemag.com/todoist-otter-ai-brainly-study-apps-adhd/

Know your brain: Default mode network. (n.d.). Neuroscientifically Challenged. https://neuroscientificallychallenged.com/posts/know-your-brain-default-mode-network

Mancuso, L., Cavuoti-Cabanillas, S., Liloia, D., Manuello, J., Buzi, G., Cauda, F., & Costa, T. (2022). Tasks activating the default mode network map multiple functional systems. *Brain Structure and Function*. https://doi.org/10.1007/s00429-022-02467-0

Orman, R. (2024, February 6). *119. default mode network vs. task positive network | how our brains balance mind wandering and focused attention - Orman physician coaching.* Orman Physician Coaching. https://roborman.com/stimulus/119-default-mode-network-vs-task-positive-network-how-our-brains-balance-mind-wandering-and-focused-attention/

Ovcharenko, J. (2024, May 9). *ADHD quotes: From sad to inspiring.* Numo ADHD.

The Pomodoro technique. (n.d.). University of Strathclyde. https://www.strath.ac.uk/workwithus/trainingconsultancy/continuousimprovementforyourorganisation/ourblogs/thepomodorotechnique/

Posner, J., Cha, J., Wang, Z., Talati, A., Warner, V., Gerber, A., Peterson, B. S., & Weissman, M. (2015). Increased default mode network connectivity in individuals at high familial risk for depression. *Neuropsychopharmacology, 41*(7), 1759–1767. https://doi.org/10.1038/npp.2015.342

Ramsøy, T. Z. (2024, August 26). *Creativity, mind-wandering, and the default mode network of the brain -.* Thomas Z Ramsoy. https://thomasramsoy.com/index.php/2024/08/26/creativity-mind-wandering-and-the-default-mode-network-of-the-brain/

Seeley, W., W. (2019). The salience network: A neural system for perceiving and responding to homeostatic demands. *The Journal of Neuroscience, 39*(50), 9878–9882. https://doi.org/10.1523/jneurosci.1138-17.2019

Seif, M., & Winston, S. (2018, April 26). *Unwanted intrusive thoughts.* Anxiety and Depression Society of America. https://adaa.org/learn-from-us/from-the-experts/blog-posts/consumer/unwanted-intrusive-thoughts

Shaw, P., Stringaris, A., Nigg, J., & Leibenluft, E. (2014). Emotion dysregulation in attention deficit hyperactivity disorder. *American Journal of Psychiatry, 171*(3), 276–293. https://doi.org/10.1176/appi.ajp.2013.130 70966

Stange, J. (2021, January 21). *Emotions in the workplace: How to deal with emotions at work.* Quantum Workplace. https://www.quantumworkplace.com/future-of-work/emotions-in-the-workplace-how-to-deal-with-emotions-at-work

Team Asana. (2024, January 29). *The Eisenhower matrix: How to prioritize your to-do list.* Asana. https://asana.com/resources/eisenhower-matrix

Torrico, T. J., & Abdijadid, S. (2019, February 10). *Neuroanatomy, limbic system.* National Library of Medicine; StatPearls Publishing. https://www.ncbi.nlm.nih.gov/books/NBK538491/

Vagus nerve stimulation. (n.d.). Wim Hof Method.

What is the limbic system?. (2024, April 6). Cleveland Clinic. https://my.clevelandclinic.org/health/body/limbic-system

Wilens, T. E., Biederman, J., Faraone, S. V., Martelon, M., Westerberg, D., & Spencer, T. J. (2009). Presenting ADHD symptoms, subtypes, and comorbid disorders in clinically referred adults with ADHD. *The Journal of Clinical Psychiatry, 70*(11), 1557–1562. https://doi.org/10.4088/jcp.08m04785pur

Yin, W., Li, T., Mucha, P. J., Cohen, J. R., Zhu, H., Zhu, Z., & Lin, W. (2022). Altered neural flexibility in children with attention-deficit/hyper-activity disorder. *Molecular Psychiatry*, *27*(11), 4673–4679. https://doi.org/10.1038/s41380-022-01706-4

ALSO BY AMY HARPER

OVERCOMING ADULT ADHD CHALENGES SERIES

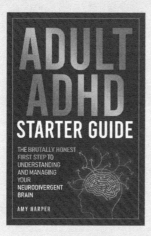

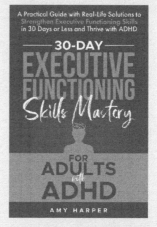

OVERCOMING ADULT ADHD CHALLENGES

Visit Amazon's Overcoming Adult ADHD Challenges Page and shop for all books. Check out pictures, author information, and reviews for the series.

SCAN ME

Made in the USA
Monee, IL
30 June 2025

20309573R00104